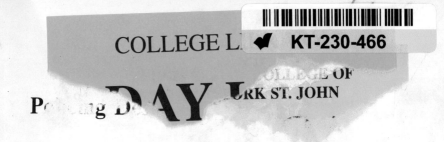

Media & Society
Richard Bolton, series editor

POLICING DESIRE

PORNOGRAPHY, AIDS AND THE MEDIA

by Simon Watney

A Comedia book
published by Methuen

A Comedia book
first published in 1987 by
Methuen & Co. Ltd
11 New Fetter Lane, London EC4P 4EE

© *1987 Simon Watney*

Typeset by Photosetting, 6 Foundry House, Stars Lane,
Yeovil, Somerset.
Printed in Great Britain by
Unwin Bros, The Gresham Press,
Old Woking, Surrey

British Library Cataloguing in Publication Data
Watney, Simon
Policing desire: pornography, AIDS and the media,
1. AIDS (Disease) – Social aspects
I. Title
362.1'042   RC607.A26

ISBN 1-85178-022-X
ISBN 1-85178-023-8 Pbk

Cover design by Richard Doust

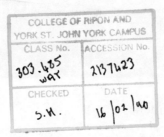

Contents

Acknowledgements   v

Introduction   1

1   Sex, diversity and disease   7

2   Infectious desires   22

3   Moral panics   38

4   Aids, pornography and law   58

5   Aids and the press   77

6   Aids on television   98

7   Safer representations   123

8   Epilogue   136

Notes   149

Suggestions for further reading   155

Index   157

For C.A.B.

Acknowledgements

I would like to thank a number of people who have been especially helpful and supportive to me in the process of preparing and writing this book. Help has ranged from a bottle of wine to newspaper clippings, from long evenings of discussion to telephoned reminders to set the video recorder for yet another Aids documentary ordeal. So, thank you one and all to Peter Aggleton, Keith Alcorn, Dennis Altman, Jennifer Batchelor, Beverley Brown, Angela Carter, Emmanuel Cooper, Russell Cullen, Mark Finch, Alison Hennegan, Hilary Homans, Meurig Horton, Dr Simon Mansfield, Mandy Merck, David Rampton, Peter Scott, Jo Spence, Jeffrey Weeks and Kaye Wellings.

I have delivered early drafts of parts of the book as lectures at the Universities of Birmingham, Edinburgh and Reading, at the Bristol Watershed Media Centre, and at Middlesex Polytechnic and the Polytechnic of Central London, where I teach. I would like to thank everyone involved in organising these talks, and all those who contributed to discussions at the time. I would also like to thank my boy friend John-Paul for his patience and steady encouragement throughout, and my editor at Comedia, Russell Southwood, who backed the project in the first place.

My largest debt of gratitude, however, must go to three dear and loyal friends in the United States, who have literally kept me posted over the last three years about developments throughout America, providing an endless flow of cuttings, newspapers, slides and magazines. My gratitude and love to Charles Barber, Jan Grover and Lisa Zeiger.

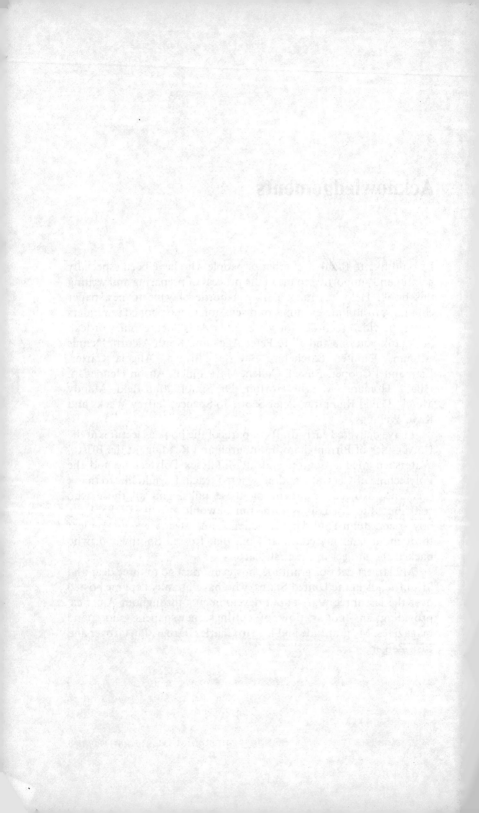

Introduction

Turning the pages of my Sunday newspaper recently, I came across a photograph of a man pushing another man's head down into a large bucket. Over the edge of the bucket emerges a pair of rubber gloves, like something struggling to clamber out. In the background there is one sign which reads "Gents Hairdresser", and another, hand-written on a piece of paper pinned up above the bucket – which reads "Free Head Dip". The accompanying article by Robin McKie is entitled "Aids scare is unkindest cut", and the caption immediately underneath the picture says simply "Lucky dip: Alan Cresswell disinfects a customer".[1]

From the article I learned that Mr Cresswell "has found an unusual way to promote his barber's business in Tewkesbury, Gloucestershire. He has placed a dustbin full of disinfectant outside his shop and asked all customers to stick their heads in it". The local newspaper had apparently run a story about measures announced by local health officials to halt the spread of Aids through the use of infected barbers' scissors. McKie reports the words of the environmental health officer involved, saying that "it's all got out of hand ... We only wanted to change regulations governing sterilisation of instruments at acupuncturists and ear-piercers so that they covered hairdressers as well. It was a precautionary measure for the future. There's no Aids in Tewkesbury." He added: "This has been sensationalised by the local press." Then Dr Anthony Pinching from St Mary's Hospital in London is called in to deliver the *coup de grâce* to the story, explaining that "provided a barber's shop implements the standard hygiene measures that have been in common practice for decades, there is no danger of picking up the virus from scissors or razors".

Elsewhere in the same edition of the *Observer*, generally held to be the only "serious" Sunday newspaper left in Britain, I read a much briefer piece under the heading "AIDS Challenge", which described how nurses at Prince Charles Hospital, Merthyr Tydfil "are threatening to take legal action against Mid-Glamorgan Health

Authority if it fails to inform them when they are treating Aids victims. They complain that an Aids patient now at the hospital is being nursed by staff who were told only that they were dealing with 'a highly contagious case'."

Now the *Observer* and Mr McKie, its Science Correspondent, might argue that by drawing attention to the situation in a small country town they are effectively helping to defuse an otherwise ridiculous situation resulting from press sensationalism. I am not convinced by such "explanations". Nor am I convinced by the words of the environmental officer that there is "no Aids in Tewkesbury". Still less am I convinced that such journalism contributes anything more than a sense of confused bewilderment to most readers. None of the thousands of people touched by this epidemic in Britain would take it so lightly. And particularly so in the context of the Welsh report, with its casual talk of "Aids victims" and the uncorrected assumption that Aids is a contagious condition, requiring extra-ordinary preventative measures in hospitals. If nurses are this worried, how is the rest of the population supposed to feel? What about the situation of people with Aids living in the community – how will other people react to them, and how will they react to their illness? These are not questions that concern the *Observer*, which is quite content to peddle the same kind of trash on the subject of Aids as any of its "gutter press" rivals, from which it purports to hold itself aloof.

A number of important points need at once to be established. Firstly, we must distinguish between a viral infection of the blood, HTLV3, or HIV (Human Immunodeficiency Virus) as it is now officially described, which attacks and may destroy the body's immune system, and is not contagious; and Acquired Immune Deficiency Syndrome (Aids) which is the collective name given to a very wide range of opportunistic infections which follow in the train of the virus, as a result of the body's weakened self-defences. Many of these are cancers and tumours that are not themselves infectious. As Professor Pinching points out in the *Observer*, standard hygiene regulations already in force are more than adequate to the task of preventing the accidental spread of the HIV virus. Yet events and stories like this continue to proliferate at a galloping pace. Newspapers like the *Observer* regularly exploit the irrational anxieties on which they are based, failing almost invariably to behave responsibly or with any compassion whatsoever for the situation of the two million or so gay men, scattered throughout the UK, whose lives have been irrevocably affected by this epidemic and who are supporting friends and loved ones through the by now grimly familiar routines of protracted illness, funerals and mourning, in a situation of acute permanent anxiety and stress. Somewhere in *The Great Gatsby* Scott Fitzgerald observed that there is no distinction so absolute as that between the sick and the well. Whilst no illness can be shared, it may, however, be relieved. Fighting Aids is not just a medical struggle, it involves our understanding of the words and images which load the virus down with such a dismal cargo of appalling connotations.

From very early on in the history of the epidemic, Aids has been mobilised to a prior agenda of issues concerning the kind of society we wish to inhabit. These include most of the shibboleths of contemporary "familial" politics, including anti-abortion and anti-gay positions. It is therefore impossible to isolate the representation of Aids, or campaigns on behalf of people with Aids, from this contingent set of values and debates. Aids is effectively being used as a pretext throughout the West to "justify" calls for increasing legislation and regulation of those who are considered to be socially unacceptable.

Homosexuality has long been at the receiving end of such campaigns. It was in a similar climate that the modern gay identity was harassed into existence in the first place. Why homosexuality should be so vehemently targeted in this manner constitutes one of the central themes of this book. In a culture which is as thoroughly and pervasively homophobic as ours, Aids can only too easily undermine the confidence and very identity of many gay men. It may equally, however, have the opposite effect, arousing intense anger against the institutions which so brutally and callously disregard the enormity of this crisis as it is being lived through, day after day, by those most directly involved in it. As one of the finest commentators on the subject, Richard Goldstein, has observed, in the context of predictions that perhaps one in ten of gay men in New York City will contract Aids: "Straight folk seem like tourists, oblivious to the blitz".[2] Should I need to spell it out, that would mean 200,000 deaths in New York alone, 100,000 in London.

At this moment in time it is impossible to know how many people would agree with the words of Rabbi Julia Neuberger that "it is a strange God who chooses to punish male homosexuals and not female, and who is angry with drug-takers who inject intravenously but not with those who sniff".[3] We must also consider the almost total blanketing of information about the emotional and psychological consequences of having tested positive to the virus' antibodies, the terrible stress in thousands and tens of thousands of gay relationships, let alone the experience of having Aids itself. Sympathy goes to mothers and children, to haemophiliacs and those who contracted Aids through blood transfusions which were contaminated before the virus was even isolated. But for gay men with Aids there seems nothing but hatred, fear, and thinly veiled contempt. The British media cares as much about our health as *Der Sturm* cared about that of the Jews in the 1930s. This is especially wicked, since gay people with Aids have to deal with a situation in which there is little hope of a cure, and they cannot necessarily rely on families and non-gay friends. When the possibility of re-infection feels like a continual "threat that's everywhere and nowhere", as one friend of mine with Aids describes it, the emotional resources needed in trying to repair one's immune system are all too often used up in defensive measures against the surrounding incendiaries of hysteria.

On top of the deaths of our friends, and our own fears for ourselves and those closest to us, gay men currently face a massive resurgence of militant aggressive homophobia. Six years into this epidemic the press is still able casually to imply that the HIV virus is contagious and thus catchable from casual contact, in the face of all medical research the world over. When someone repeats something which they know to be untrue, you can fairly take one of two explanations. Either the person is deliberately lying, or else they are incapable of recognising the truth. I believe that most Aids commentary on television and in the press falls into the second class. For this reason we need to attend particularly closely to the voices which talk most publicly of Aids. In this book I am attempting to do just that – to listen carefully to what I have described elsewhere as "the rhetoric of Aids".[4] I have attempted to analyse the overall discursive structure of Aids commentary, paying special attention to its repetitions, its slippages, its omissions, its emphases, its "no-go" areas, its narrative patterns, and so on. I have not set out to cover every aspect of this commentary, and have not tried to draw a chart of how different groups of people with Aids have been categorised. Least of all have I tried to write a "history" of the epidemic. For England alone, that would be an encylopaedic task. Nor have I shied away from using terms which may be unfamiliar for some readers, though I have tried carefully to define them as and when they arise. Simple language cannot always explain complex phenomena. You would not try to cut through welded steel with plastic knives and forks.

This is a book about representation, written in the belief that representation is not merely a reflection of "real life", but an integral part of it. In times of crisis we can see cultures concentrating on themselves, and their profiles are telling. From the fierce heat of hysteria a dim light is generated against which we may sometimes make out an inkling of the future. Whilst there is no necessary connection between the current situation in which gay men find ourselves, and different oppressions affecting other social groups, I hope that this book will make at least a small contribution to the larger process of understanding the workings of power and oppression. Whilst we owe it to our friends with Aids to give them all the love and support we can, we must also help them by directing our gaze away to those who have made their situation so intolerable. But we cannot challenge them unless we are confident in ourselves, individually and collectively. As gay activist and attorney John Wahl argues:

> "We need to become aware of our own worth, and that means absolutely dumping the mental and psychological restraints we have adopted ... [from] ... a culture that puts down same-sex affection and makes us very cautious ... You have to absolutely never accept second class humanity or second class citizenship for any reason whatsoever, not even for tactical reasons."[5]

We must also attend to the question of what we can and need to do, as asked and answered by Ben Schatz, the Director of the National Gay Rights Advocates (NGRA) Aids Civil Rights Project in America:

> "First, we have to come out – and not just to those we think will be supportive, but to those whose rejection we fear most. That means coming out to grandma, whose feelings you've been trying to spare while she votes to have you quarantined ... We have to start being pushier with our apathetic gay and lesbian friends and get them involved. Next time someone tells you they need their space, tell them they won't have much space if they're quarantined."[6]

In such ways Aids can make us strong.

Originally this book was to be illustrated, but the newspapers involved ignored requests for permission to reproduce material. The *Observer* inexplicably refused to give permission to reproduce the photograph referred to on page 1.

Chapter One

Sex, diversity and disease

In January, 1986, I lost a friend to Aids. I weigh these words carefully, as I weigh my sense of loss, and my motives for writing this book. My friend did not die "of Aids", but from one of the many opportunistic infections to which the body is prey when its defensive immune system has been extensively damaged. As the writer Iris Murdoch, whom he much admired, has observed:

> "The careful responsible skilful use of words is our highest instrument of thought and one of our highest modes of being: an idea which might seem obvious but is not now by any means universally accepted."[1]

Bruno died in France, in hospital, with his father who had looked after him in his last few weeks of life. He had not contacted anyone from his old circle of close gay friends in England. His funeral took place in an ancient Norman church on the outskirts of London. No mention was made of Aids. Bruno had died, bravely, of an unspecified disease. In the congregation of some forty people there were two other gay men besides myself, both of whom had been his lover. They had been far closer to Bruno than anyone else present, except his parents. Yet their grief had to be contained within the confines of manly acceptability. The irony of the difference between the suffocating life of the suburbs where we found ourselves, and our knowledge of the world in which Bruno had actually lived, as a magnificently affirmative and life-enhancing gay man, was all but unbearable. After the funeral we all retired to his parents' home, a group of relatives and old friends. It was evident that whilst his mother and father had been able, in private, to accept Bruno's sexual identity, they could not begin to handle the enormity, as they saw it, of Aids. They were thus unable to share his death either with their relatives or nearest friends. Least of all could they share their grief with their next-door-neighbours. They were afraid. Not of a virus, but of a scandal more terrible even than the fact of homosexuality. They had been condemned to silence. to euphemism, to the shame of guilt by association, in this the most devastating moment of their lives as parents. I was, of course, deeply moved and shaken by their plight, and decided there and then that I would write a book on the subject of

Aids. Not a medical book, but one which would try to make some kind of sense of what had been done to these people.

My friend was not called Bruno. His father asked me not to use his real name. And so the anonymity is complete. The garrulous babble of commentary on Aids constructs yet another "victim". It is this babble which is my subject matter, the cacophony of voices which sounds through every institution of our society on the subject of Aids – the voices of doctors, priests, teachers, politicians, newsreaders, journalists, lawyers, feminists, nurses, firemen, children, actors and, out on the very fringes of social audibility, the voices of people with Aids (PWAs) themselves.

Four months after Bruno's death the Centers for Disease Control in the United States announced that 20,000 Americans had been diagnosed with Aids. Of these, nearly 11,000 were already dead. In Britain, as I write, there have been approximately 900 cases, of whom, as elsewhere, more than half have died. No ordinary calculus of grief can measure the worldwide map of tragedy and loss and anger on the part of those directly touched by the catastrophe. Yet this catastrophe is unique, in that it has been systematically denied the status of either tragedy or natural disaster for the vast majority of those it most immediately affects. We are all victimised by the discourse of "victims" which dominates the entire social profile of Aids, a discourse characterised by an initial and enormously significant reversal whereby, as Jeffrey Weeks has pointed out, most people with Aids are themselves blamed for the illness.[2]

It is a commonplace of medical history that every epidemic proceeds from an initially vulnerable community. The HIV virus has manifested itself in three constituencies which are already feared and marginalised in the West – blacks, intravenous drug-users, and gay men. The presence of Aids in these groups is generally perceived not as accidental but as a symbolic extension of some imagined inner essence of being, manifesting itself as disease. Further, in different ways for all three groups, Aids has been used to articulate profound social fears and anxieties, in a dense web of racism, patriotism and homophobia. It is this web, spun out in words sticky with blood lust, contempt, hatred, and hysteria, which hangs across the entire media industry of the Western world, and beyond.

This, then, will be a book about representation, written from the belief that we can only ultimately conceive of ourselves and one another in relation to the circulation of available images in any given society. As Richard Dyer writes:

> "A major legacy of the social political movements of the Sixties and Seventies has been the realisation of the importance of representation. The political chances of

different groups in society – powerful or weak, central or marginal – are crucially affected by how they are represented, whether in legal and parliamentary discourse, in educational practices, or in the arts. The mass media in particular have a crucial role to play, because they are a centralised source of definitions of what people are like in any given society. How a particular group is represented determines in a very real sense what it can do in society."[3]

Such an attitude may be widely held within the specialised realm of contemporary Media Studies, but it has still hardly touched wider political constituencies, where television and newspaper images are generally assumed to reflect, or misrepresent, the "truth" of the world. I write from the assumption that there is not in fact a single, unified "truth" about Aids, available to be represented directly and universally or, for that matter, to be misrepresented. Rather, I hope to show some of the ways in which a particular virus, one of the simplest life forms on the planet, has been used by a wide variety of groups to articulate a host of issues and concerns, consciously and unconsciously. Although the overall effect may be that of some deafening chorus, I hope to demonstrate that many different and frequently conflicting positions have been struggling for ascendancy.

It is clear that Aids has unleashed at least as many currents of thought and prejudice among lesbians and gay men as elsewhere. I have recently, for example, discovered in the middle of a well-argued and highly theoretical essay on Safer Sex techniques, the statement that "at this point in the twentieth century ... gay men do not have time for theory, we only have time for practice".[4] I can do no more than strongly disagree with any such conclusion. Now, more than ever, we need to understand clearly and precisely what forces and values are mobilising in relation to the ongoing crisis of Aids. For Aids is not only a medical crisis on an unparalleled scale, it involves a crisis of representation itself, a crisis over the entire framing of knowledge about the human body and its capacities for sexual pleasure. This is why we should resist any temptation to jump to immediate conspiracy theory explanations for the press or television industry's coverage of Aids. We will not be able to understand what is being said, and to whom, in such messages until we have considered the larger and prior assumption that newspapers and television address a uniform and exclusively heterosexual "general public". Nor could the most exhaustive and systematic sociological and economic account of the media explain the uneven rhetoric of Aids as it is spoken across the media.

Somehow we have to be able to account for the voice of the information officer of a South London borough who refuses to allow any literature about Aids to be distributed within the local black community on the grounds that this is a "white" colonial illness. We have equally to account for the ritual denunciations of "promiscuity" by some Christian fundamentalists and not others, and by some gay men and not others. It is in the face of this kind of complexity that I have been drawn towards the vocabulary and methodology of psychoanalysis in my own readings of the vast Aids litter surrounding us. As Jacqueline Rose has argued, it

> "directs its attention to what cannot be spoken in what is actually said. It starts from the assumption that there is a difficulty in language, that in speaking to others we might be speaking against ourselves, or at least against that part of ourselves which would rather remain unspoken."[5]

I am writing, then, from the assumption that newspaper journalists and television script-writers invariably say more than they intend, and that the notion of intentionality – that we all know what we are saying, why we are saying it, and to whom – is profoundly unhelpful to the task of unpicking the rhetoric of Aids. We may, however, put that same rhetoric to unauthorised usage, to reveal aspects of the communications industry which are rarely discussed, to launch counter-offensives against its terms and its values.

One implication of a conspiracy theory approach to the subject of Aids and the media, of the widespread belief that a few straightforward and deliberate lies can be replaced by "the truth", is that a simple change of personnel in any given institution would be sufficient for all to be well. This seems to me to be akin to saying that nuclear energy would be "safe" if we only had the right officials at the Department of Energy. How we individually think of Aids, and respond to it, depends on our own relationship to our own sexuality – at least in so far as Aids is endlessly and inaccurately read as a veneral disease, like syphilis or gonorrhoea, rather than the result of a blood disease. The practice of HIV testing in STD clinics only serves to reinforce the highly misleading notion that Aids is *intrinsically* sexual. As Allan Brandt points out, "social values continue to define the sexually transmitted disease as uniquely sinful – indeed, to transform disease into an indication of moral decay".[6] This in turn only encourages the kinds of victim-blaming and moralising types of health education strategies which have never proved to be successful. As Brandt argues, "more creative and sophisticated approaches to this set of diseases are necessary . . . Moreover, we must recognise that behavioural change does not mean encouraging celibacy, heterosexuality, or morality; rather, it means developing means to avoid coming into contact with a pathogen".[7] The early classification of

Aids as an STD has undoubtedly encouraged the widespread articulation and distribution of powerful *non-medical* meanings by which the HIV virus has been effectively colonised.

In this sense at least, we can think of misrepresentation in the limited sense of incorrect information about the HIV virus, its molecular structure, modes of transmission and so on. Yet, even in the most obscure medical journals, we will not find pure clinical "facts", since medicine, like any other professionalised branch of knowledge, is invariably informed by social and historical context. When the very word "disease" is itself so potent a metaphor, we cannot expect individual diseases to be entirely metaphor-free. If Aids is to be a metaphor for anything, it is up to us to make sure that in time it becomes regarded as a glaring example of how the ill may be victimised far beyond their physical symptoms, and of how far a deeply racist and sexist society will go to prosecute its own ends.

Three years ago in New York I read a now notorious article by Larry Kramer, casually, in a friend's apartment. Like many others, I dismissed it angrily at the time as wild scare-mongering of the worst kind:

> "If this article doesn't scare the shit out of you we're in real trouble. If this article doesn't rouse you to anger, fury, rage, and action, gay men have no future on this earth. Our continued existence depends on just how angry you can get."[8]

My anger was self-defensive, and I failed to note the call to mobilise, in hope, alongside the outraged anguish. Coming back to London I forgot all about it. The same friend wrote to me two years later about the situation in New York:

> "Life staggers on, the morning newspaper horrors making the outside world seem unreal and several galaxies away. It's like being punched very hard in the stomach. Petty worries and anxieties – how will I earn any money this summer, etc. – become doll-sized suddenly, but equally vital because private. Complaining about *anything*, however, becomes ridiculous: we who have everything. 'Are you happy?' 'I'm alive & fed & unbombed – yes.' But that won't tell you anything about me. You asked me about AIDS – said I rarely mention it. Well, what is there to say? It's a horror, too... I participated in a series of four hour interviews for the Columbia Medical School Public Health AIDS Project – gay-run of course... I came of sexual age fully believing... that freedom meant multiple partners – I really did (and do)

believe it. Now we have to rethink that from a health point of view without abandoning sex (which most are doing in theory if not in practice). I went out to Boybar Saturday night, the first time 'out' in ages – but a deep chill came over me – hard to describe but I felt physically lonely . . . and that's the wrong, I mean, a too-desperate way to go out . . . it screams from a mile away. I couldn't be there lightly, and didn't want to be there with this desperate need, so I left! Home on the faithful bicycle. A lot of men seem to consider blatant cruising passé now, and disgusting. This is very unfortunate – if anything, we should be having more (safe) sex not less. NYC has been more or less useless for AIDS patients, San Francisco much better. My friend Tim's brother in SF had all of the symptoms, and to such a terrible degree, that he called his friends and family together to his apartment, they had dinner, and he said good-bye and took several handfuls of sleeping-pills with coffee and dessert. He lay down to sleep while they sat with him."

What is at stake here is a fundamental issue of identification. In Britain Aids is viewed almost exclusively from the heterosexual viewpoint, which offers speaking roles to other heterosexual PWAs but never to the constituency most devastated by the disease. Our newspaper and television reports consistently refuse any identification *with* gay men under any circumstances. The gay man is effectively and efficiently positioned as he-with-whom-identification-is-forbidden. There is thus no possibility in Britain for the framing of Aids as anything other than a "gay plague", (a phrase still widely in use in the British press), as if the syndrome were a direct function of a particular sexual act – sodomy – and, by extension, of homosexual desire in all its forms. Thus, by contingency, even lesbians are suspect and newly newsworthy. The entire discourse of Aids turns round the rhetorical figure of "promiscuity", as if all non-gays were either monogamous or celibate and, more culpably still, as if Aids were related to sex in a quantitative rather than qualitative way. Clearly journalists know that their readers are unlikely to be effortlessly monogamous or celibate, so we must conclude that the term "promiscuity" is being employed to other purposes – as a sign of homosexuality itself, of forbidden pleasures, of *threat*. What we read is a literature of containment, endlessly policing human sexuality, as if the powers of the police themselves were insufficient to contain the dangers of deviance, henceforth to be branded indelibly with the ideological skull-and-crossbones sign of Aids. Just as menstruation was used for centuries as "evidence" of Fallen Eve in every woman, so Aids is recruited as the natural, just and due reward for sex outside marriage.

Yet, as an American commentator pointed out in 1983:

> "fidelity can never be regarded as a measure of commitment when it is inspired by the threat of illness; celibacy as an alternative to death is a painful, numbing choice."[9]

And in reply to an admonishing friend who asks, "Why can't you people just fuck less?" offers,

> "No easy answer, except to suggest that for many gay men, fucking satisfies a constellation of needs that are dealt with in straight society outside the arena of sex. For gay men, sex, that most powerful implement of attachment and arousal, is also an agent of communion, replacing an often hostile family and even shaping politics. It represents an ecstatic break with years of glances and guises, the furtive past we left behind. Straight people have no comparable experience, though it may seem so in memory. They are never called upon to deny desire, only to defer its consummation."

He concludes that,

> "for heterosexuals to act as if AIDS were a threat to everyone demeans the anxiety of gay men who really are at risk, and for gay men to act as if we're all going to die demeans the anguish of those who are actually ill..."[10]

Journalism of such an exceptionally high order is indicative of a society in which the negative, guilt-ridden homosexual of the 1950s and 1960s has largely given way to the sex-affirmative gay culture of all the major American cities. It is also indicative of a publishing industry not subject to the British obscenity and indecency legislation, which has guaranteed, until the summer of 1986, that all the leading American gay newspapers and journals (containing the only alternative to the frothing and gibbering of our local mass media) have been entirely illegal. Hence, for example, the almost incredible yet typically British story of how the chief medical officer at the Department of Health had to have copies of *The Advocate* and *New York Native* quite literally smuggled into England in diplomatic bags, in order to avoid seizure by British customs officials, whilst the government's public information campaign on Aids was being drawn up.[11] There is not the least possibility in contemporary Britain of anything remotely resembling the celebrated "L.A. Cares – like a mother" campaign in Los Angeles, which addressed gay men as one community amongst many in the city, offering a phone number for

Safer Sex advice on giant hoardings and on television.

In the short term there might seem to be possible benefits from the displacement of attention away from actual gay PWAs and on to the larger perceived threat to the community, from which we, as gay men, are needless to say excluded. In this respect the erasure of the homosexual from the field of British social life as anything other than a miscreant or criminal, functions somewhat paradoxically at present to prevent certain more blatant forms of scapegoating. But this would be a very short-sighted view indeed, since it overlooks the fact that in Britain the very existence of a positively-identified gay community has gone almost entirely unnoticed by the state and media alike. In effect, British gay men live out their lives in a culture which continues to think of and represent them as "homosexuals", with all the most advanced medical and psychiatric connotations of the late nineteenth century. Indeed, one of the most unfortunate aspects of the media coverage of Aids in Britain has been the gigantic opportunity it has afforded most commentators to treat the two words "homosexual" and "gay" as if they were synonyms, as if gay liberation and the entire Sexual Politics movement of the 1970s had simply never happened.

But, in any case, British gay politics has lacked that powerful ideal and model of Civil Rights which is so centrally inscribed within the American constitution and Bill of Rights. As Dennis Altman has written:

> "The development of a sense of gay identity is a phe-
> nomenon peculiar to America, where the tendency to
> perceive oneself as part of a group rather than a class
> underlies the whole liberal notion of politics and society. (In
> this, America differs from a number of European and Latin
> American societies, in which class and ideology are
> considered much more significant and where, accordingly, it
> is less easy to develop the idea of one's sexuality as a basis for
> social and political identity.) On the other hand, the
> acceptance of group diversity in America has always existed
> within very severe limits... to the extent that they are
> prepared to subscribe to the dominant values of the society;
> to go outside these values is to be denounced as un-
> American."[12]

We can fairly discern a situation of relative advantage and disadvantage between American and British gay men. Since the 1950s, Supreme Court rulings have tended to protect the position of gay publications in America in the name of "freedom of speech" in ways which are unthinkable in the United Kingdom, where only one licensed shop has survived recent legislative purges to sell the mildest forms of sexually explicit gay materials and sex-aids (known in a characteristically more friendly and positive way in the United States as "toys") – dildos, leather wear and so on. Yet at the same time American gay culture has conspicuously failed to develop the types of collectivist institutions, organised neither for profit nor for sexual exploitation, which abound in Britain in the form of co-operatively owned cafes, discos, information switchboard services, legal organisations and publishing houses, as well as a flourishing tradition of independent gay theatre, pop music, film, poetry, and fiction, which is clearly at odds with dominant cultural values and institutions. For this there is little or no equivalent in the United States, where collectivism appears decidedly un-American.

Such social and cultural differences count for little, however, with magnates such as Rupert Murdoch, whose international media juggernaut is scarcely aware of, or at all concerned for, the niceties of national, let alone regional or sexual variations of readership. Newspapers, like commercial television, are produced to sell advertising space. There is little point in wasting time at this end of the century in regrets for what we have lost in the possibility of a media industry constructed on behalf of a diverse community of actual viewers, rather than an abstract "general public", flattered and flattened into broad bands of potential purchasing power. Yet the precise mechanisms of how gay men and lesbians are regarded in and by this industry remains an important question, and one which has been signally and significantly overlooked in all previous accounts of the media, right across the political spectrum. The initial question here is not why homosexuality is stigmatised as such, but why it is made so consistently to seem extraordinary, something quite out of the way of everyday social life, something no newspaper reader or television viewer might reasonably be supposed to think about under any decent circumstances. This is a question which I shall come on to consider in much greater detail.

One of the greatest ironies of the Aids epidemic has been the way in which the interests of gay men have been ignored, by and large, both by the far left, but also by the middle-ground of British and American party politics. Aids has only been extensively taken up as a political issue in both countries by the far right, ever eager to discover new threats to the apparently endlessly vulnerable values of hearth and home. In this respect Aids has been used quite cynically to shore up the fabric of the ideology of patriotic heterosexuality. Whilst Reagan and Thatcher wage real wars on imaginary external aggressors (Nicaragua, the Malvinas islands, Grenada, Outer Space), another ideological spearhead is being launched against an enemy within. Not a virus which can and must be conquered but rather those who suffer from it, premised as the sexually promiscuous, and with them, by extension, all other enemies of "the family", the sacred and largely imaginary locus of neo-conservatism in all its variant forms and voices. In the ever anxious neo-conservative imagination, the family sits, a familiar thing, rather like the small, homely valley town of a 1950s B-movie, nestling a couple of miles downstream and out of sight from the towering dam which (as our hero and heroine and their 2.8 children snuggle down chastely after prayers in pyjamas under granny's patchwork quilt) we see to be on the very point of imminent collapse.

But such horror of sex, and of homosexuality in particular, should not automatically be dismissed as "sham" moral repugnance, or hypocrisy. For the roots of sexual anxiety reach down deep beneath our culture, and burrow under all formal social divisions of class, gender, race, age, sexuality, religion, and explicit political alignments. Such anxiety is always, ultimately, seated in the human body itself, and our attitudes to our own bodies and one another's. As Michel Foucault has argued:

> "The body is directly involved in a political field; power relations have an immediate hold upon it: they invest it, train it, torture it, force it to carry out tasks, to perform ceremonies and to emit signs. The political investment of the body is bound up, in accordance with complex, reciprocal relations, with its economic use; it is largely as a force of production that the body is invested with power and domination; but, on the other hand, its constitution as labour power is possible only if it is caught up in a system of subjection... the body becomes a useful force only if it is both a productive body and a subjugated body."[13]

All the major institutions and industries of society crowd round us constantly to subjugate our bodies – in the various names of health, beauty, strength, masculinity, fashion, motherliness, respectability and so on and so forth. Their exhortations are always to some extent in mutual conflict, and nowhere more so than in relation to our sexuality, where, for example, notions of modesty or decency may in some circumstances be aligned with notions of the glamorous and the desirable, whilst at other times they are opposed, recruiting us to rival and incompatible attitudes to ourselves. In this manner divisions in the social world may be experienced as painful divisions within the self, leading to a rejection of the weaker voice, and retrenchment around the stronger. Hence, the situation in contemporary feminism, where many women are tugged back into a culture of very traditional femininity in the name of "dignity" or "self-respect", terms which other feminists will read as powerful agencies of repression. The ways in which we respond to such exhortations can never be reduced simply to our class origins, or race or nationality, but to the complex psychic history of the individual as it negotiates these categories. Hence the seemingly bizarre alliances in contemporary Britain and America between neo-conservatism and the women's movement, a subject to which again I shall return in some detail.

The ways in which gay men are able to organise in relation to Aids – both to the medical and the ideological situation, is dependent on our image of ourselves, and this imagery is always and everywhere subject to state intervention and control. This is nowhere more apparent than in contemporary Britain, where as recently as August, 1985, charges were brought against a London bookshop, Gay's The Word, under the Customs and Excise Consolidation Act of 1876, concerning almost 150 books, including works by Jean Genet, Allan Ginsberg, Edmund White, Tennessee Williams, Kate Millett, Jean Paul Sartre, and Oscar Wilde... That all charges were dropped in June, 1986, is only due to the perseverence of the bookshop and its defence campaign, and the recognition that British law is out of step with European Community statutes. In this case, as in so many others, it is clear that the state's prosecuting position was profoundly muddled and confused. A medical book on Aids was seized alongside Boyd McDonald's *Straight To Hell* "true homosexual experience" anthologies. What matters in such instances is that we defend the latter as vigorously as the former, and do not collude with a censorship system which evidently regards all references to homosexuality as such to be intrinsically indecent and/or obscene. The Gay's The Word case also involved copies of France's *Gai Pied* as well as the *New York Native*, which has consequently been unavailable in London since the original police raids early in 1984. If I did not have good friends in the United States I would have had no possible means of access to any of the most serious debates concerning the politics of Aids and the media, the recent Lyndon Larouche initiative in California, and so on. Censorship sets a *cordon sanitaire* around lesbians and gay men in Britain, a barrier which has guaranteed a major standstill in the development of a broadly-based, affirmative gay culture in Britain. As Dennis Altman recognised in the early 1980s,

"the risk to gay identity seems greater in countries such as Great Britain and the Irish Republic, where the gay movement has less legitimacy and seems less able to withstand a new ideological onslaught, backed by real fears and dangers."[14]

We are now facing that onslaught in relation to Aids, which threatens not only our health but our very social identity, as the term "gay", wrenched away from the older pejorative discourse of "homosexuality", is reloaded before our very eyes with all the familiar connotations of effeminacy, contagion and degeneracy. Gay culture in the 1970s offered the grounds for the emergence of a social identity defined not by notions of sexual "essence", but in oppositional relation to the institutions and discourses of medicine, the law, education, housing and welfare policy, and so on. As such it has been strikingly successful across the field of discourse. It has also enabled, as I have suggested, the development of a wide variety of cultural forms and social formations, in relation to which at least two generations of young people whose sexuality is predominantly homosexual have "come out" into a previously unimaginable social identity. It is this new and fragile (if confident) gay identity which is now particularly at risk, not from Aids as such, but from the crisis of representation surrounding it. This new gay identity was constructed through multiple encounters, shifts of sexual identification, actings out, cultural reinforcements, and a plurality of opportunity (at least in large urban areas) for desublimating the inherited sexual guilt of a grotesquely homophobic society.

By encouraging a wholesale de-sexualisation of gay culture and experience, Aids is now proving a significant obstacle to this process. We are already witnessing an ominous "re-homosexualisation" of homosexuality back into a culture of repression which, I should add, is the antithesis not of sexual "liberation" but of sexual affirmation.[15] Thus, whilst individuals are vulnerable to HIV infection, the entire reproductive machinery of gay subjectivity is also vulnerable to the ideological fall-out of the representational crisis triggered by the virus. Nor is this only the case in Britain. The recent report of the American Meese Commission on "pornography" clearly recommends "a repressive agenda for controlling sexual images and texts: vigorous enforcement of existing obscenity laws and the passage of draconian new measures."[16] Calls for increased sexual censorship across the United States in recent months share the same spurious appeal to defensive measures against Aids, and even on behalf of PWAs themselves. Thus Victor Cline, speaking on the subject of pornography at a conference held in Boston in November, 1985, on "Morality in The Media", argued that "pornography exposure lessens taboos and leads to sexual aggression, multiple partners and deviance. Pornography leads to multiple partners which, if conditions are right, may lead to Aids." Other speakers also focused on supposedly "irresponsible" gay men, and the presumed connections between pornography and Aids. One doctor presented a slide show, like those used by anti-abortion and anti-porn campaigners supposedly to demonstrate the iniquity and appalling effects of their chosen targets. He showed a large number of images of active cases of syphilis, gonorrhoea, and herpes, finishing up with opportunistic Aids conditions including Kaposi's sarcoma. His aim was clearly to associate Aids with venereal disease, in a narrative of moral outrage and physical disgust.

It is in this climate that we must become increasingly sensitive to the significance of debates within our own local gay communities, and to the agenda which they establish. The editorial in a recent American gay sex magazine baldly states that,

> "Discretion is an asset. Let's face the facts. It's no longer cool to be gay. Not any more. The days of the screaming queen are in the past, or should be ... Why wave the fag-flag in their faces when you no longer hold the winning hand? It's time to be discreet ... Just quit being such a flighty dick-pig, bath house queen, indiscreet butt-chaser and uncontrollable whore."[17]

This is the tone and stance of any extreme fundamentalist Bible-basher, dressed up as Safer Sex advice and, as *The Body Politic* has pointed out, is no more and no less than a gay-speak version of the dominant Aids-as-divine-retribution arguments of both secular and Christian populist moralism.[18]

More dangerous still, because more subtle, is a series of arguments which have also surfaced recently in America. Thus we find Michael Halberstadt professing that,

> "while I, for one, have clung tenaciously to the counter-cultural *weltanschauung*, much of the so-called 'gay community' veered in the direction of a clone culture, which celebrated, rather than battled, anomie. Mustachioed machos mincing in their tight jeans, cynically pursuing anonymous sex and worldly advancement ... made a parody of love and liberation."

He resents the fact that,

> "these gutless wonders now repudiate – or acquiesce in the destruction of – a liberation that, at best, they failed to grasp in the first place"

whilst at the same time he asserts the right to a time when it will

> "be safe to fuck and (if indeed it isn't) to suck again."

His article ends with a rousing declaration that,

"the Bible Belt isn't America. It can be isolated, as much as we have thus far allowed it to isolate us."[19]

Halberstadt laments the loss of a unified gay identity which, given the injuries of race and class and nationalism, as well as the sheer diversity of homosexual desire and sexual behaviour, could never be more than, at best, a projective fantasy advanced for strategic purposes – for example, the initial recruitment to gay liberation, from which noble, pure, and uncontaminated height he evidently looks down on the failures of his contemporaries. Love is opposed to sex, liberation to "worldly advancement", in a discourse which rings down the centuries, smug, holier-than-thou.

In a similar vein, Wayne C. Olson inveighs against the idea of gay politics as such, in favour of personal struggle to achieve a positive identity, as if there were not objective structures all around him making any such wish quite preposterous. Olsen "struggles" with his sexuality as he "struggles" with his weight. Both are equally conceived as problems:

"Those who advocate gay as the only way are dead wrong.
There is much validity in other kinds of sexual expression.
Why get hung up on just one thing, sexual or otherwise?"[20]

Whilst one could hardly accuse him of offering a sophisticated argument, that is not the point. What matters is the way he unconsciously reverses the fact that it is a normatively heterosexual society which denies the validity of gay sexuality, and persists in regarding it as some kind of "false copulation" (like the mating of male wasps with certain species of orchids), rather than as one fundamental and universal variant of human sexuality. In the same issue of *New York Native* Joseph Puccia offers yet another version of the same position, casting doubt on whether American society is worth entering legitimately anyway:

"Let's go underground and protect ourselves from the poisoning light of day, where joining the mainstream will dilute our feelings and destroy our culture."

His calls for "private" clubs and businesses and gymnasia are uttered with the familiar breathtaking arrogance of the (presumably) white metropolitan male, who is purblind to the fact that the vast majority of homosexual acts take place between men who have little or no choice but to be "underground" already, where homosexuality has always existed, and to where the massed forces of familial ideologues would like to consign us all once more. Looking down from his safe, complacent New York eyrie, Puccia seems oblivious to the fact that gay men are routinely persecuted and imprisoned all around the world, including his own native America.[21] Olsen wants to integrate *into* straight society, Puccia wants to stand in total autonomy *from* it. Both, however, deny the specificity of gay culture, and the extraordinary complexity of its socio-historical position. And both remain incapable of thinking through any aspect of the diversity, or mutability, of sexual desire.

Such utterances are worth attending to, however, since they illustrate so clearly the dangers of gay men falling back into an essentialist attitude to themselves and one another, as if there were indeed some "natural" and unitary essence of homosexual desire and identity, from which all variants are deviations. This is to lose sight of the diversity of homosexuality which, for Freud, as Jeffrey Weeks reminds us, "was not a single condition, but more a grouping of different activities, needs and desires."[22] Sex,

> "far from being the most natural element in social life, the most resistant to cultural moulding... is perhaps one of the most susceptible to organisation... Moreover, the forces that shape and mould the erotic possibilities of the body vary from society to society."[23]

And, of course, within them. It is the power to expand or to limit our understanding of these possibilities which constitutes the central theme of this book. Where is the agenda set which offers us our sense of who we are in relation to other positions within the sexual spectrum? How are gay men responding to the steady miniaturisation of the public perception of homosexuality? How do non-gays perceive homosexuality at a time when the word "gay" is already at least half-way to becoming a euphemism for "deadly", and the older metaphors of sickness and contagion have been all but replaced by a discourse of fatality, with Aids widely regarded as a syndrome of voluntary, deserved collective self-annihilation – the long awaited and oft prophesied spectacle of the degenerates finally burning themselves out.

Chapter Two

Infectious desires

With characteristic acuteness, Gayle Rubin has noted how,

"it is precisely at times such as these, when we live with the
possibility of unthinkable destruction, that people are likely
to become dangerously crazy about sexuality. Contemporary conflicts over sexual values and erotic conduct have
much in common with the religious disputes of earlier
centuries. They acquire immense symbolic weight. Disputes
over sexual behaviour often become the vehicles for
displacing social anxieties, and discharging their attendant
emotional intensity."[1]

This book is concerned with precisely such "discharges", with the
ways in which Aids is made to seem to speak on behalf of various
social groups, whose moral opinions thus ostensibly emanate from
the syndrome itself. It is important to unmask such feats of
ideological ventriloquism, since this is the only way in which we can
identify the individual positions which speak across the huge,
bellowing amphitheatre of Aids commentary. This amphitheatre
takes many forms; it is at once a television studio and a bar, a
newsagent's shop and the operating theatre of a teaching hospital.
One factor is common to all: the figure of the patient, who is speaking
but cannot be heard for the hubbub which surrounds him. He is
completely ignored, the person with Aids, as he-with-whom-
identification-is-forbidden. In this respect he is confined not only
within the ordinary regime of medicine, but also by the entire
apparatus of modern sexuality, both of which are continually
monitoring and controlling the public *meaning* of his illness, as
closely as his presenting symptoms.

The overall narrative structure within which Aids is almost
invariably described is not, of itself, especially interesting. Any newly
identified and seriously life-threatening disease will be discussed in
terms of its source of origin, its modes of transmission, its
recognisable signs, its range of infection, and the possibility of cure
and preventative vaccination. In the case of Aids, however, this
narrative has been massively inflected and distorted by a number of
external determining factors. Principal among these is the felt

connection between the disease itself and the social groups in which it has initially emerged, in particular gay men. Maurice Blanchot has written that "if it weren't for prisons, we should know that we are already in prison".[2] In this respect the gay man is always in any case a prisoner, aware that behind him there stretches out the long shadow of "the homosexual", for signs of which parents anxiously scrutinise their uncomprehending offspring, and against whom they literally and metaphorically double-bolt the nursery windows night after night. Two major streams of images and their related associations converge to constitute this shadow. Firstly, the notion of homosexuality as a contagious condition, invisible and always threatening to reveal itself where least expected. And secondly, the spectacle of erotic seduction, in which "innocent", "vulnerable" youth is fantasised as an unwilling partner to acts which, nonetheless, have the power to transform his (or her) entire being. Thus I read in the sex education textbook which was in my school library in the 1960s that it is,

> "obvious that sexual love among persons of the same sex is a perversion because, quite apart from any other arguments based upon ethics and morality, such a practice cannot result in procreation... The greatest danger in homosexuality lies in the introduction of normal people to it. An act which will produce nothing but disgust in a normal individual may quite easily become more acceptable, until the time arrives when the normal person by full acceptance of the abnormal act becomes a pervert too."[3]

There is an important internal conflict at work within this text, and countless like it, concerning the "normal" person's "disgust", and the seeming ease with which it is apparently over-ridden. If this were the case, and one accepted a contagion/seduction model of homosexuality, then everyone would be at risk from pleasures which remain too awful and dangerously seductive for the text to dwell on... It needs to be understood that the widespread association of homosexuality with the subject of child molestation is not accidental, but stems from the way in which homosexuality has been theorised since the late nineteenth century, when the word largely replaced other terms and produced the idea of a single, coherent, uniform type of human being – "the homosexual". As I have written elsewhere,

> "on the one hand there was the invert, the 'natural' (e.g., incurable) homosexual, emotionally and/or physically attracted to his own sex. And on the other there was the 'passive' and, it was generally assumed, basically hetero-

sexual object of the invert's desires. Homosexuality was thus theorised from its very conception as a relation between predatory seducers and (their) 'innocent' victims. What is at stake here are the ways in which the invert/pervert hypothesis has been transmitted through the mass media of the twentieth century, the ways in which homosexuality has been regarded as 'newsworthy' and hence given a particular public profile... which constitutes the prevailing commonsense on the whole subject."[4]

It is the long cultural legacy of this body of belief, hearsay and superstition which continues to posit "the homosexual" as the subject rather than the object of victimisation. The reality is that homosexual desire is not triggered from nowhere by the vile attentions of older seducers, perverts who lead young heterosexuals into lives of unspeakable depravity. On the contrary, most gay men will look back to their childhoods as a time of hopelessly unfulfilled emotional and physical frustration, sunk, as Edmund White has put it so graphically, "into a cross-eyed, nose-picking turpitude of shame and self-loathing".[5] There can be few so privately lonely in the modern world as the homosexual child. Hence the need to insist on non-natural explanations of sexuality, and to follow through Freud's argument that it is the fixity of sexual choice of any kind, whether for the same or the opposite sex, or both, which deserves attention, rather than the object of desire itself.[6] For it is only by unravelling the complex inheritance of a theory of sexuality which carves up humanity into two vast and immutable camps that we can hope to get to grips with the full significance of contemporary Aids commentary. In this manner we can begin to draw up useful maps of the incomparably strange ideological spaces in which lesbians and gay men are obliged to live out our lives. However knowing and sceptical we may be concerning the immediate archaeology of our own identities – increasingly understanding more about the conditions of emergence of the modern binary categories of sexuality – we nonetheless have to recognise ourselves both in terms of a "homosexuality" constructed at the interstices of laws about the age of consent, immigration, taxation, property, parenting and so on, as well as in our own culture, which bears so very little resemblance to the historical figure of "the homosexual". This figure is constituted in law, but also with equal immediacy in the entire structure of representations flowing through our "host" society.

On the one hand we are invited to think of ourselves as a coherent, unified group, roughly analogous to race, deriving from a supposedly shared and primary level of sexuality. On the other hand we actually experience our social being as a series of discontinuous exclusions through which we move at work, in our families, and elsewhere, always modified by the contingent factors of class, education, the nature of our employment, and so on. This is why the notion of belonging to a single "gay community" is ultimately unhelpful and unconvincing. For whilst we may collectively resist particular instances of injustice, campaign for the improvement of our civil liberties, and celebrate and support ourselves within a culture of sexual affirmation, this does not imply any essential unity to homosexual desire as such. We undoubtedly constitute a constituency of shared interests in relation to the workings of police, state and other institutions of power. But this should not lead us to lose sight of the diversity of human sexuality in *all* its variant forms, which it is perhaps the most radical aspect of gay culture continually to assert and expose. As a result, every gay man is always "of" yet not entirely of his ascribed social position within the triangle of class, race and nationality. His sexuality is always, by degrees, at variance with the alignments which he knows he is expected to take to the great institutions of marriage, child-raising and property, together with their myriad reflecting rites and rituals. These will "trouble" his sexuality, as he will "trouble" them, only as long as sexuality is conceived in predominantly – if not exclusively – heterosexual terms. To all intents and purposes the subject of his sexuality remains firmly locked in a discourse of "nature" which ceaselessly regards the male as predatory and the female as "naturally" preyed upon, thus erasing any question of *volition* on the part of either. It is precisely this question of sexual *choice* which is foregrounded most directly by homosexuality, which is consequently strictly confined within the framework of predatoriness, with connotations of child molestation, the corruption of "youth", and so on, or else read off as a species of gender confusion working in an opposite direction to "feminise" certain men, thus making them "unnatural". In either event the overall ideological structure is protected from the threat of a sexuality which invariably refuses the heterosexual/"nature" paradigm for thinking sex.

Here a simple anecdote might serve to help. I am drinking in a gay pub in London with some friends. Three young men appear, in their early twenties, immediately too "loud" to register as gay. They become an object of mild interest, mainly defensive, since three men can pull a good few punches before they're thrown out. As we all suspected (unspoken) two of them begin to strike peculiar poses, the postures of "queers" they've seen on television. They giggle and shriek and are having a whale of a time. By now nobody is taking any notice of them. They are unlikely to be violent. However offensive they may seem, this is tempered by a certain pathos – the sight of people who are both unaware that they appear ridiculous, and objects of silent contempt on the part of the very men (and women) whom they themselves so demonstrably despise. Despise, that is, until one of them needs to go to the lavatory. Everything changes. "Watch out John! Keep your back to the wall! Watch out for the wankers!" etc. Yet nothing has altered around them. The Janus-like figure of the "queer" has simply been turned round in their heads. A bar full of contemptible, feminised men has been invisibly transformed into a menacing crowd of sinister, powerful predators. They at last see us as we see them, but without the humour or the pity. Finally the risk of being raped proves too much for them, and they leave, reverting to heterosexuality by way of the mincing queen once more. Back at the bar they're already forgotten. Another incident averted. But the boys will talk about it for weeks, how they were all touched up, how John had his bottom pinched, how they had a good laugh, how they hardly got away with their lives.

This was perhaps a ritual purging, or a test of some kind, for the three young men involved. Who knows? The same thing happens regularly in every gay bar all over the world. Yet it is precisely in such incidents which are not "incidents" ("the police reported to-night...") which illustrate most sensibly the ligatures of sexuality in everyday life, though I very much doubt if the same men would enter a gay bar today: there is now another sign over the door in their eyes, regardless of the name of the pub. In such intimate, unhesitating and seemingly self-directed ways is the body subjugated, in their case by a life-long slipstream of words and images, in relation to which they had entered the bar in the first place and, disappointed, had performed their little pantomime of received images. It was, however, a moment in which, confronted by the terrifying, ordinary, recognisable world of homosexuality, they had been compelled to act out a necessary "Other" which would return to them their prestigious identities as "heterosexuals" intact. That, I believe, was the virginity which was threatened that night – the truly disturbing acknowledge-ment of sexual diversity within the confines of the known and the *familiar*, in which they were indistinguishable from the "queers", and momentarily perceived themselves as such.

Thus, the figure of the gay man interrupts yet also reinforces the social and psychic boundaries of desire, and the relations of gender which are inscribed within them. Straight society needs us. We are its necessary "Other". Without gays, straights are not "straight". Which is why homosexuality is so dramatically theorised as either an *absence* or an *excess* of "manliness". This is not, however, merely to conclude that homosexuality and heterosexuality sit on an even footing, locked together in mutual opposition. For the modern tendency to derive notions of social identity and individual character from sexuality works quite differently in relation to them both. Historically, "the homosexual" has been incited to think of his core essence as a perverse negative of heterosexuality, which is taken as the norm right across the major discursive fields of sociology, anthropology, psychiatry, medicine, jurisprudence, politics, education and psycho-analysis. The gay man, on the contrary, affirms his sexuality in a category which is fundamentally socio-political, and implies no intrinsic common factor with other gay men beyond the workings of power on the entire range of homosexual desire in all its variant forms, which are unified only in their collective affirmations of value and validity. This is quite different from the identity of "the heterosexual", for whom heterosexuality does not designate desire for the opposite sex, so much as a rejection and denial of homosexuality. Thus, homosexual identity involves a primary and self-abasing awareness of *not* being heterosexual, whilst heterosexual self-awareness involves an equally primary sense of *not* being homosexual. Neither term has sexual object-choice as its central meaning, unlike the category "gay", which remains a positive term of immediate collective and self identification. It thus escapes the entire frame of reference, and the power relations invested within the epistemology (or theory of knowledge) of sexuality as such, which is simultaneously produced and policed in the negative persons of "the homosexual" and "the heterosexual".

Sexuality, conceived in these terms, is inevitably brutalising for everyone caught up in its ruthlessly over-simplified categories of homo- and hetero-sexuality. In particular, it forces homosexual desire to recognise itself, and be recognised within the constricting mould of a performance-based theory of sexual and social identity, which ultimately bifurcates the entire latitude of homosexuality into two rigid subject positions, "active" and "passive", on the basis of a vulgar behaviourist reading of heterosexual sex. The psychological damage which inevitably results from the process of actually living out one's life in these terms remains incalculable for "the homosexual" and "the heterosexual" alike. As my anecdote is intended to demonstrate, both exist as co-products of discourse, prior to and directive of whatever may actually be before one's eyes. In this respect, however, it is important to remember that homosexuality can only be envisaged in our culture against the impoverished and impoverishing yardstick of a heterosexuality, the normative power of which seeks absolute hegemony. Hence the strenuous ideological work to "pull back" the category gay into the dominant orbit of the orthodox structure of sexuality, which is propped up and reinforced at every point by the institutions and discourses of the state and science in all their manifestations. The inescapable conclusion emerges that our most basic classificatory systems for making sense of sex are grossly inadequate to the task, in so far as they delimit any possible understanding of sex to a single, monolithic binary opposition. In this context, biological sex difference, and what Freud calls "object-choice",[7] may not be the correct starting points for the study of sex at all. Whether we are exclusively attracted sexually to the same or the opposite sex may be of comparatively little significance compared to the initial ways in which we come to recognise and realise the integrity of our own bodies, and other people's. In this sense we would expect to find much deeper and more elemental structures of desire underpinning the entire range of human sexual potential than can possibly be imagined, let alone theorised in the given, dominant epistemology of sex.

Turning to the field of representation, it is apparent that homosexuality, as it is currently construed, contravenes both limited codes concerning the depiction of specific acts, such as sodomy between men, as well as much larger, regulative dichotomies which are derived from the anatomical distinction male/female, the attributes of which inform the entire taxonomic field of Western logic. Above all, homosexuality problematises the casual identification of primary power with the figure of the biological male as masterful penetrator. It equally problematises the parallel identification of powerlessness and passivity with the figure of the biological female as submissive and penetrated. For the gay man is truly polymorphous: he may fuck and be fucked, and is as much at home in the one fantasy-position as the other. He does not need the defensive refuge of an identity rooted in exclusive models of domination or submission, which can never make adequate sense of his psychic and physical mobility. To the extent, however, that these models constitute the major available iconography for sexual fantasy in our society, the gay man or lesbian is endlessly able to play off such roles against one another, thus effectively exorcising them without being damaged in the process by the actual violence and hatred which are the inevitable products of sexuality and its categorical imperatives. This is why most self-defining "heterosexuals" seem more than a trifle unreal to lesbians and gay men, although, as Neil Bartlett has written: "If a gay man can see heterosexuals as delightful fictions, he must also acknowledge their real and terrible power".[8]

Nowhere does this power inhere more clearly than in the domain of public representations, since the very notion of "the general public" is massively heterosexualised, and for reasons which I shall consider in detail in my chapter on Aids reporting in the press. It goes without saying that the degree of heterosexualisation of the news media goes more or less unnoticed by most heterosexually identified viewers and readers. If the very concept of sexuality is indeed, as I have suggested, intrinsically paranoid, an initial look at British television and newspaper coverage of Aids will bear out the point more clearly still. Writing in Rupert Murdoch's increasingly far right *Sunday Times*, Liz Jobey describes the American photographer Bruce Weber's latest book, *O Rio de Janeiro*, the proceeds of which will go to New York's Aids Resource Centre. Interviewing Weber for her imaginary audience of Thatcherite zealots, Jobey sets an agenda which is standard in the British press. The Centre, she explains, "takes in Aids victims who have been rejected by their families and friends".[9] She describes Weber's work for Calvin Klein and Ralph Lauren as "overtly sexual and for the first time, but in tune with the times, revealed men as sensually provocative". Having described the book, she notes that,

> "Weber recognises no irony in his chosen cause, dismissing any suggestion that his photographs, with their almost deification of the male body, might in some way have glorified homosexuality".

What is happening in this text is both simple and complex. We are effortlessly manoeuvred from Weber's opening words, that "anyone in our business has lost friends in the last couple of years" to the spectre of "Aids Victims", and from there to the question of male bodies, perceived as "sensually provocative". What is unstated but crucial is the transgressive possibility that men might find one another's bodies "provocative", even – horror of horrors – to the point of being sexually desirable! It is this ghastly possibility from which it is evidently Liz Jobey's job to protect the average male *Sunday Times* reader. Hence the remotest notion that one might be sexually affirmative about male homosexuality is made to seem both extraordinary in itself, and morally questionable. What is being said between the lines is that homosexuality "causes" Aids, and therefore anything to do with the subject must be handled with surgical rather than the conventional kid gloves.

A couple of weeks earlier the main *Nine O'clock News* on BBC1 television[10] included a major item on the subject of Aids, announced by an unseen male presenter's voice informing us that "doctors say Aids could affect every family in Britain", the same unproblematically heterosexual family unit which is so clearly the locus point for the editors and journalists who produce the news. Now seen beneath an enlarged colour image of a white-coated scientist gazing earnestly into a laboratory microscope, the reporter continues:

"The disease Aids could be killing more than 400 people a month in Britain within five years according to doctors, and the British Medical Association warned today that it could affect anyone who is sexually active. The report goes on to say that prevention is not just better than cure – it is the only cure."

These closing words are flashed up on to the screen, beneath a picture of the *British Medical Journal* issue from which the "story" derives. The image of the peering scientist then fills the screen, moving into motion to give tracking shots of faceless technicians fiddling purposefully with any amount of high-tech gadgetry, and close-ups of impressively incomprehensible computer print-outs, as the voice-over continues:

"Doctors say up to 40,000 people in Britain carry the Aids virus, most without knowing. Of nearly 400 identified cases here, half have died. Four years ago the Americans also had 400 cases, now they have got 20,000 and at least 1,000,000 are infected."

This last sentence is read out over a graphic showing first the Union Jack, and then the British flag entwined with the Stars and Stripes, with a large caption, "The AIDS Problem", and the statistics reported. The voice-over carries on:

"Unless a treatment is found, it is predicted that 180,000 Americans will die in the next five years. With Britain following the same pattern, it is anticipated that by then, deaths in this country will be equivalent to the crash of a fully loaded jumbo jet every month."

This latter point is fortunately not illustrated. "Doctors say it's not just a homosexual problem. Anyone with more than one partner is at risk."

We then cut to Charles Farthing, who is described as an "AIDS specialist", and informs us that "I feel that by the end of the century there won't be one family in the UK that isn't touched in some way by this disease, either by the loss of a brother or a sister, relative or friend." We then cut again, this time to Dr John Dawson from the BMA seated in an interview studio:

–   Dr Dawson, can we be clear? Aids is in the heterosexual community now. What sort of heterosexual is at risk?

–   If men and women are having sex with more than one partner, if they are promiscuous, having sex with several partners, then there is a risk, not only of catching Aids, but of transmitting it to other people. Now this is the way in which Aids is caused – you don't catch it by being sneezed on or by normal social contact, in an office or in a shop or a school. You get it from intercourse, and it's no longer homosexual intercourse, it is heterosexual intercourse that can give it to you, and other things like intravenous drug abuse.

– So that means promiscuous, casual sex can be a killer?

– There is that risk, and as time goes on the risk will increase, because there is no prospect of any vaccine or cure for Aids in sight, and the way not to get Aids is to restrain your sexual activities in that sense.

– Is that message being put across strongly enough do you think?

– We don't think so, because we're not seeing the changes in public behaviour that will control the disease in this country, and we do think that a much greater effort is needed by government, to get the message out much more clearly so that we can emulate San Francisco, for example, where the disease appears to be controlled in this way, rather than New York, where they're failing to control it.

– Dr Dawson, thank you very much.

What on earth are we to make of this heady brew of lip-smacking innuendo and plain misinformation, much of which is dangerous in the extreme, validated by the full institutional authority both of the BMA and the BBC? What is initially so offensive is the script-writer's patent inability to comprehend just how many families are already affected by Aids in Britain. But since gay men are perceived through the ideological filter of "homosexuality" they cannot be acknowledged as parts of families. The implication remains that we need to take Aids seriously now that it's no longer just killing off the queers ... Hence the peculiar phrasing used by Charles Farthing, whose picture of the family "at risk" significantly desexualises the parents by omission. What is being protected here is a fantasy on the part of the news concerning its actual viewers, who have been hectored into the assumption that it is sex *per se* which "causes" Aids, since there is no recommendation to enquire of prospective sexual partners whether they are gay, or bisexual, or IV drug-users, or whether they have had sex lately with members of these groups. That at least would have been of some use. Instead, Dr Dawson merely goes on and on about the alleged risks from "promiscuity", regardless of the fact that one can contract Aids if one has only had one sexual partner in one's entire life. The number of sexual partners one has is completely and totally irrelevant to the subject of HIV infection. What does matter, and which wasn't even mentioned here, was the question of the type of sex one has, and the need to use condoms. This last point is absolutely crucial, and the *BBC News* report was positively counter-productive. All we are left with is the familiar complacent critique of the promiscuous, those supposedly outside families, viewed from the largely imaginary perspective of the television audience as a set of regular family units – mum and dad sitting on either side of the fireplace with the children in bed ... the national British family as it is routinely addressed by the *BBC News*. Above all, this national family unit must not be shocked or upset in its own living rooms by the mention of actual sexual behaviour. Unable to discuss the realities of sex in an adult manner, the television audience is simply infantilised, and told to give up sex altogether, like smoking or anything else that is incontrovertibly "bad for you". This is about as irresponsible as it is possible for television to be. "Not just a homosexual problem" indeed ...

My final general example of the heterosexualisation of the news media is taken more or less at random from the current issue, as I write, of *Working Woman*.[11] It is the cover story – "AIDS – NO ESCAPE: Expert Report" – alongside a full page photograph of a woman and man kissing with their eyes open, both tinted blue. The illustration also serves to anchor features on Italian design, the Inner London Education Authority, careers in languages, and Italian fashion. The magazine's editor, Pandora Wodehouse, writes in her monthly Editor's Letter that "AIDS should not be considered a predominantly homosexual disease – our feature tells you why, and what we can do to prevent it spreading". Three points immediately spring to mind. To begin with, Ms Wodehouse takes for granted that we think of Aids, or any other disease for that matter, as obedient to the unstable structure of Western theories of sexuality. Implicitly, Aids is seen to have been until recently a "homosexual disease", whatever that might be. Secondly, the "we" to whom she writes, which is a female "we", evidently does not include the possibility of lesbian readers, since if the disease is no longer "homosexual" and in consequence now threatens "us", "we" cannot be homosexual ourselves. Thirdly, there is the implicit narrative suggestion that Aids becomes feature-worthy only when it threatens the readers of *Working Woman*, who apparently cannot possibly know or care about anyone who has developed the syndrome in the last four years. Aids should never be referred to as if it were an attribute of any social group as such. It is a complex medical syndrome, not a property of persons.

We then move on to the article itself, "AIDS – Who's Next?" by Robin McKie, the "expert" referred to on the cover, and Science Correspondent of the *Observer*, whom we have already come across. As so often in journalism, individual writers hawk their wares around, so that the press is in effect endlessly talking to itself in a series of internal correspondences. The cover photograph is reproduced again at full page size, but this time with some overlayed artwork removed to show that the woman is naked at least to the waist, whilst the man wears a loose sweater of sorts. In the meantime, however, the dark tone of their skin and hair has been coloured red, as if they were somehow irradiating from within. I cannot help finding unfortunate and misleading connotations here of the possibility of infection by casual contact, in the air, like radiation ... This quite apart from the vexed question of kissing, to which we will have frequent occasion to return.

McKie's story begins with a description of June,

> "a fifty-three year-old mother of two. With her grey hair pulled back in a bun, and matronly clothes, she is a perfect image of middle-class respectability. Yet June has con-tracted AIDS. The very antithesis of a victim of a disease that most British people associate with promiscuous homosexuality, June has succumbed to an ailment that is now spreading alarmingly across the world."

Like many other people with Aids, June has actually succumbed here to British journalism, being used as a kind of ideological glove-puppet behind which McKie can introduce his position, having set the initial scene. June is middle-aged, middle-class, presumably white (or her race would be mentioned), and assumed without question to be a heterosexual as a mother of two. Above all, she is "respectable". She is not, as far as we know, promiscuous. She embodies the notion of the "innocent victim" in the media rhetoric of Aids, the blameless person who has contracted Aids as a direct result of someone else's perfidy, the "guilty victims" – the queers, the blacks, the junkies, and the prostitutes.

"At present," McKie goes on, "only a few British women have contracted Aids. Nevertheless, doctors say that numbers will soon rise as a bridging group of bisexuals and drug-takers begin to spread the disease to the female population". The female population is, of course, a subject of anxious attention to (presumably) heterosexual journalists, since it is from this direction that they evidently think themselves to be at increasing risk, thus "blaming" women as vectors of disease, just as Victorian prostitutes were blamed as contaminated vessels, conveyancing "female" venereal diseases to "innocent" men, and just as gay men are blamed today for spreading a "homosexual" disease to "innocent" heterosexuals. Having talked about prostitutes in Edinburgh who have been infected by their drug-using boyfriends, McKie moves on, since,

> "drug takers are not the only ones who pose danger to women. Bisexuals are also a threat. 'One in three of the homosexuals we see in our clinic are Aids virus carriers,' says Professor Michael Adler of London's Middlesex Hospital. 'In addition, about ten per cent of gays are also bisexual. That means that a considerable number of men must now be passing on the virus to women.'"

There are at least three substantial points which need to be made here. Firstly, it is apparent that a by-now familiar reverse-discourse is in complete control of the narration, ensuring that our attention is not distracted to the position of people with Aids in the "guilty victim" categories, understood as homogenous totalities. Secondly, an ideological valve seems to be at work, which only admits discussion of risks to potential "innocent victims" through on to the surface of the printed page. At the same time, I very much doubt whether Professor Adler used the actual words ascribed to him, since he has always been punctilious in his rejection of such obfuscating terms as the "Aids virus". How many times does one have to inform a professional science correspondent, who has already had the temerity to publish one not very helpful book on the subject, that people with Aids are only "victims" of predatory journalists, and that it does not clarify medical matters endlessly to collapse the issue of HIV virus infection – a blood disease affecting the body's immune defence system – into the symptoms of individual opportunistic infections which result from severe damage to the body's immunological defences. Idle talk of an "Aids virus" is at best misleading and at worst culpably mischievous. Lastly, we can detect the severe problems which innocent reporters encounter when confronted by the actual diversity of human sexual behaviour. The immediate instinctive tendency to line up with the "respectable", to disavow the very existence of sexual wishes or behaviours which do not immediately match up with the public profile of the Royal Family, is perhaps the most significant aspect of the British news media's coverage of the entire epidemic.

At least McKie does spell out clearly that,

> "despite all the insinuations of the popular press, Aids is still difficult to contract; the Aids virus [sic] is only transmitted through the interchange of bodily fluids – blood, semen and

vaginal secretion – so danger comes from having sex with an infected person of either sex. To be ignorant of this risk is to put oneself in danger."

The implication here seems to be that ignorance itself is a voluntary state, and culpable. In any case, this leads directly into the article's major argument, supported by "Aids experts in America", against "casual sexual encounters". A London doctor is introduced to modify this somewhat with the caution that "if they feel they must – and we are all humans after all – they should insist that men wear condoms and should also use spermicides". The main problem, however, is evidently "promiscuity", with issues about the kinds of sex one has pushed firmly into the background. The entire discourse feeds into a moralistic rejection of "fast lane" sex, and the implication, always mobilised around female sexuality, that sex *per se* is intrinsically dangerous. McKie then turns, after his fashion, to the situation of the person with Aids:

> "Although being diagnosed an Aids virus carrier is certainly not a death sentence, it still brings much anguish. Carriers are unlikely to get life insurance, may fail to get mortgages, may lose their jobs and face a lifetime of sexual isolation (for the Aids virus is believed to linger in the body and brain for ever)."

This is about as near as "serious" journalism gets to acknowledging the existence of PWAs, rather than the "threat" which they are made to pose to the rest of humanity. It is not an edifying picture. All that McKie sees is Homo Economicus, struck down on the battlefield of career prospects and property. Not a word is said about the injustice and possible illegality of such examples of outrageous discrimination, nor is there the slightest flicker of concern for the devastating psychological consequences of this epidemic for the entire gay population of Britain, regardless of their individual HIV antibody standing.

"For women," McKie continues, "the position is, if anything, worse. Doctors now strongly advise that female virus carriers avoid pregnancy and even recommend abortions to those already carrying unborn children." It would seem that the pivot of human values exists on an axis involving parenting to the exclusion of all other factors. Motherhood is the goal of womanhood. Why should any other aspect of a woman's life concern us, or her? Anonymous doctors once more shake their heads at us from the page, in a mime-show of abstract medical authority, interrupting the text in order to back up McKie's moralism on a firm foundation of "science". This is followed by a great deal of general information about Aids, describing how,

> "the virus... spreads throughout the body eventually crippling the immune system. Aids victims are then left powerless to fight a range of normally innocuous microbes. As a result, they succumb to the effects of these viruses, bacteria and tumours. Victims have an average survival period of eighteen months."

All the person with Aids has to do is to sit back and wait to die, according to this prescription. Fortunately we are all able, at the very least, to fight back against this kind of journalism, with its banal marshalling of "average" periods of life expectancy, and its completely fatalistic collusion with orthodox medicine. There is no serious discussion of immunology as such, let alone any advice on how those with impaired immune systems – across a wide range of medical conditions – might be able to help themselves.

The article ends with a coda of source-hunting, with monkeys a familiar and well-tried point of departure in the virus' mission to wipe out blacks, gay men, the "promiscuous" and – by extension – sex in any non-reproductive sense. McKie ends, sensibly enough, with the inescapable conclusion that only "explicit health education pro-grammes can stop the disease's spread", education which his own article misses another opportunity to provide. A final doctor is introduced in order to impress the point that people

> "must be told explicitly what are the dangers of picking up the Aids virus. And when we do so, we have to shock people with our terminology. We can no longer afford to worry about offending people's sensibilities. There are too many lives at stake for that."

But not too many, it seems, for *Working Woman* and McKie, who leave the good doctor huffing and puffing away bravely to nobody, since whatever he had to say that is so terribly "shocking" is left far, far out of hearing on some untranscribed cassette. This is especially important, since the question of just how Aids is being discussed in schools, or could be, might have provided the opportunity for a really useful article, in the place of this tired old mess of re-heated mass media cliché. If anything about the coverage of Aids is "shocking" it is this preposterous posturing on the part of "experts" who claim to be about to deliver up the last word on the subject, the dreadful "Truth", for which publishers and editors of magazines like *Working Woman*, and programmes like the BBC's *Nine O'clock News* are continually exhorting us to brace ourselves.

As I have already suggested, there is no single universal "truth" about Aids, or any other disease for that matter. What Aids actually

dreadfully vulnerable to other people's disease. Thus, commentary produces expectations, and expectations fan out into lived experience.

> "An eighteen year-old Coventry man, who thought he had caught Aids after drinking from the same bottle as a gay man, punched and killed him, Warwick Crown Court heard on Friday."

The man received a three-months sentence in this "wholly exceptional case".[3] "Theatre cleaners are threatening to boycott a group of gay actors because they are frightened of catching Aids".[4] Such stories are invariably accompanied by denials that Aids can be contracted via casual contact, but their framing is always top heavy, focusing on fear rather than allaying it, dramatising anxiety rather than alleviating it.

The most widely favoured explanation amongst lesbian and gay commentators of the social climate surrounding Aids lies in the theory of moral panics. Drawing on the influential school of "new" criminology from the 1960s, which tried to explain the social context of crime and "deviance", Stanley Cohen described in 1972 how societies

> "appear to be subject, every now and then, to periods of moral panic. A condition, episode, person or groups of persons emerges to become defined as a threat to societal values and interests; its nature is presented in a stylised and stereotypical fashion by the mass media; the moral barricades are manned by editors, bishops, politicians and other right-thinking people;... Sometimes the panic passes over and is forgotten, except in folk-lore and collective memory; at other times it has more serious and long-lasting repercussions and might produce such changes as those in legal and social policy or even in the way that society perceives itself."[5]

For Cohen the mass media provides "a main source of information about the normative contours of a society...about the boundaries beyond which one should not venture and about the shapes the devil can assume."[6] The mass media is understood to construct "pseudo-events" according to the dictates of an unwritten moral agenda which constitutes newsworthiness. Thus "rumour... substitutes for news when institutional channels fail",[7] and in ambiguous situations "rumours should be viewed not as forms of distorted or pathological communication: they make sociological sense as co-operative improvisations, attempts to reach a meaningful collective interpretation of what happened by pooling available resources."[8]

Subsequent writers such as Stuart Hall have opened up this debate about the representational strategies behind different types of moral panic, arguing that they are indicative of how people are persuaded "to experience and respond to contradictory developments in ways which make the operation of state power legitimate, credible and consensual. To put it crudely, the 'moral panic' appears to us to be one of the principal forms of ideological consciousness by means of which a 'silent majority' is won over to the support of increasingly coercive measures on the part of the state, and lends its legitimacy to a 'more than usual' exercise of control".[9] Hall's work on the historical structures of British racism has encouraged him to develop a "stages" theory of moral panics, leading to ever increasing punitive state control (although he would be the first to admit that it is not only the state which is involved, however loosely we may define it). This is equally a problem for anyone trying to analyse the representation of homosexuality in terms of available theories of moral panic, since the entire subject is historically constituted as "scandal", with subsequent calls for state intervention.

In an important essay on Aids, Jeffrey Weeks relies heavily on moral panic theory, explaining how its mechanisms

> "are well known: the definition of a threat to a particular event (a youthful 'riot', a sexual scandal); the stereotyping of the main characters in the mass media as particular species of monsters (the prostitute as 'fallen woman', the paedophile as 'child molester'); a spiralling escalation of the perceived threat, leading to a taking up of absolutist positions and the manning of moral barricades; the emergence of an imaginary solution – in tougher laws, moral isolation, a symbolic court action; followed by the subsidence of the anxiety, with its victims left to endure the new proscription, social climate and legal penalties."[10]

Gayle Rubin also sees special "political moments" in the history of sexuality, observing that,

> "moral panics rarely alleviate any real problem, because they are aimed at chimeras ... They draw on the pre-existing discursive structure which invents victims in order to justify treating 'vices' as 'crimes' ... Even when activity is acknowledged to be harmless, it may be banned because it is alleged to 'lead' to something ostensibly worse ..."[11]

Dennis Altman also discusses Aids in terms of moral panic, but modifies the notion against local and national factors. Thus, "the

Australian panic is not only a product of homophobia but is also tied to the ... belief that they can insulate themselves from the rest of the world through rigid immigration and quarantine laws" and "a less sophisticated understanding and acceptance of homosexuality than exists in the United States".[12] Calls for draconian legislation in such disparate societies as West Germany and even Sweden, lead him to conclude that "the link between Aids and homosexuality has the potential for unleashing panic and persecution in almost every society."[13]

Whilst such analyses offer a certain descriptive likeness to events, they also reveal many severe limitations, which suggest the inadequacy of the concept of moral panic to the overall ideological policing of sexuality, especially in matters of representation. To begin with, it may be employed to characterise *all* conflicts in the public domain where scape-goating takes place. It cannot, however, discriminate between either different orders or degrees of moral panic. Nor can it explain why certain types of events are especially privileged in this way. Above all, it lacks any capacity to explain the endless "overhead" narrative of such phenomena, as one "panic" gives way to another, or one anxiety is displaced across different "panics". Thus one moral panic may have a relatively limited frame of reference, whilst another is heavily over-determined, just as a whole range of panics may share a single core meaning whilst others operate in tandem to construct a larger overall meaning which is only partially present in any one of its individual "motifs". Clearly there is not (yet) a moral panic in British or American government circles, compared to their public profiles over, for example, immigration, pornography or abortion. But this is only to say that the theory of moral panics makes it extremely difficult to compare press hysteria and government inaction, which may well turn out to be closely related. In both instances we are facing symptoms – symptoms of sexual repression which manifest themselves across a spectrum which ranges from stammering embarrassment to prurience, hysterical modesty, voyeurism and a wide variety of phobic responses. In other words, the theory of moral panics is unable to conceptualise the mass media as an industry which is intrinsically involved with *excess*, with a voracious appetite and capacity for substitutions, displacements, repetitions and signifying absences. Moral panic theory is always obliged in the final instance to refer and contrast "representation" to the arbitration of "the real", and is hence unable to develop a full theory concerning the operations of ideology within all representational systems. Moral panics seem to appear and disappear, as if representation were not the site of *permanent* ideological struggle over the meaning of signs. A particular "moral panic" merely marks the site of the current front-line in such struggles. We do not in fact witness the unfolding of discontinuous and discrete "moral panics", but rather the mobility of ideological confrontation across the entire field of public representations, and in particular those handling and evaluating the meanings of the human body, where rival and incompatible forces and values are involved in a ceaseless struggle to define supposedly universal "human" truths.

What we are dealing with in such phenomena is the public forum in which modern societies and individuals make sense of themselves. Together with the increasing industrialisation of this forum, we should note its centrality for political debates where interest groups attempt to bypass the traditional structures of democratic process in order to force the enactment of laws in the name of the "good" of a population which is never actually consulted. This is precisely what the mass media were invented to do, since they have evidently never responded to the actual diversity of the societies which they purport to service. We are looking at the circulation of symbols, of the basic raw materials from which human subjectivity is constructed. It is not in the least surprising that those attempting to manipulate conscious attitudes should play on themes which possess deeper, unconscious resonances. Hence the danger of thinking of newspapers or television as being primarily concerned with "news" values, as distinct from entertainment, or drama, or sports coverage, or advertising, or whatever. For all these categories of production share an identical presumption about their audience, which is projected across them in different genres as a unified "general public" over and above the divisions of class, age and gender. This subject audience is massively worked on to think of itself in the terms which familiarity has established through repetition. The very existence of homosexual desire, let alone gay identities, are only admitted to the frame of mass media representations in densely coded forms, which protect the "general public" from any threat of potential destabilisation. This is the context in which we should think about the crisis of representation with which Aids threatens the mass media, understood above all else as an agency of collective fantasy. Aids commentary does not "make" gay men into monsters, for homosexuality is, and always has been, constructed as intrinsically monstrous within the entire system of heavily over-determined images inside which notions of "decency", "human nature" and so on are mobilised and relayed throughout the internal circuitry of the mass media marketplace.

It is the central ideological business of the communications industry to retail ready-made pictures of "human" identity, and thus recruit individual consumers to identify with them in a fantasy of collective mutual complementarity. Whole sections of society, however, cannot be contained within this project, since they refuse to dissolve into the larger mutualities required of them. Hence the position, in particular, though in different ways, of both blacks and gay men, who are made to stand outside the "general public", inevitably appearing as threats to its internal cohesion. This cohesion is not "natural", but the result of the media industry's modes of address – targeting an imaginary national family unit which is both white and heterosexual. All apparent threats to this key object of individual identification will be subject to the kinds of treatment which Cohen and his followers describe as moral panics. What matters is to be able to understand which specific groups emerge as threats to which "societal values and interests". Moral panics do not speak to a "silent majority" which is simply "out there", waiting to listen. Rather, they provide the raw materials, in the form of words and images, of those moral constituencies with which individual subjects are encouraged to identify their deepest interests and their very core of being. But in so far as these categories are primarily defensive, in so far as they work to protect the individual from a partially perceived threat of diversity and conflict, they are also themselves vulnerable. Hence the repetition of moral panics, their fundamentally *serial* nature, the infinite variety of tone and posture which they can assume. The successful policing of desire requires that we think of "the enemy" everywhere, and at all times. This is why there is such a marked conflict throughout the entire dimension of Aids commentary between the actual situation of people with Aids, and the model of contagion which they are made to embody.

We are not, in fact, living through a distinct, coherent and progressing "moral panic" about Aids. Rather, we are witnessing the latest variation in the spectacle of the defensive ideological rearguard action which has been mounted on behalf of "the family" for more than a century. The very categorisation of sexuality which I described in Chapter One is part of this same action. How we respond to it is therefore of the greatest importance, since at this point in time our liberties and very lives are being put increasingly at risk. We need precisely to be able to *relate* phenomena which present themselves, in terms of the theory of moral panics, as discrete and unconnected. Thus we may draw a significant parallel, for example, between local American state decisions to enact laws which refuse confidentiality to those who have tested positive to HIV infection (despite the clear advice and recommendation of the Centers for Disease Control that confidentiality should be a priority), and the recent decision of British police to arrest the singer Boy George at the clinic where he was being treated for heroin addiction. In both instances a "moral" agenda has permitted punitive actions which are positively counter-productive, both to limiting the spread of Aids and helping drug addicts. On the one hand, few if any gay men are likely to undertake a test which might immediately render them liable to the loss of civil liberties if the results are not kept confidential and, on the other hand – as George's doctor pointed out – retroactive charges for the past possession of drugs are unlikely to encourage addicts to come forward for treatment.[14] The *Village Voice* reported in May, 1986, that since the state of Colarado introduced identification record requirements for people wanting HIV tests, applications at gay men's health clinics have dropped by 600 per cent in only three months. In both cases actual practice at local state and police levels flies in the face of clearly stated medical and governmental policies. Both cases also illustrate the danger of identifying individual "moral panics" in a simple one-to-one relation to their ostensible targets. This is why I prefer to think in terms of Aids commentary, rather than assuming the existence of a unified and univocal "moral panic" over Aids.

A similar problem occurs if we try to explain away all the variations and nuances of Aids commentary as epiphenomena deriving from a single source. This, however, is very frequently the case, and the source most readily identified by lesbians and gay men is "homophobia". This is hardly surprising when *The New York Times* feels sufficiently at liberty to print a long article by the American darling of the New Right, William F. Buckley, which concludes, after acres of drifting around, that,

> "everyone detected with AIDS should be tatooed in the upper fore-arm, to protect common-needle users, and on the buttocks, to prevent the victimisation of other homo-sexuals."[15]

The last time people were forcibly tattooed was under Nazi rule, when millions were slaughtered because their politics or race or sexuality, or combinations of these, did not conform to the master plan of a totalitarian state. Such prescriptions remain unthinkable in relation to any other category of American citizen. But Buckley clearly regards gay men as so far "outside" the body politic that no measure is too extreme to contemplate. What is so very remarkable about such pronouncements, however, is that they are announced *on behalf* of gay men and, at the same time, are "balanced" on the same page of the newspaper in question by another article which eloquently insists that "those who have a stake in using AIDS to prove the morality or immorality of any particular lifestyle, should be deemed disqualified from the scientific debate."[16] This may, in some respects, be naive, since presumably all scientists subscribe to some system of moral judgement or another; nonetheless, as the writer points out, "the flow of solid data should not be polluted by personal moralism".

In Britain last June (1985), the *Times* gave its editorial space over to one Digby Anderson whose headline blazened "No moral panic – that's the problem".[17] Anderson begins where he intends to end, with an inflammatory invitation. "Excuse me, may I have the pleasure, would you care to panic?". Aids, he notes,

> "is causing considerable consternation among sexually and politically progressive persons, as well it might. But the prime cause of concern is not the threat of incurable illness and death of persons progressive or otherwise. The major matter for concern is that the consternation of non-progressive persons about Aids may inconvenience 'the gay community' and damage progressive efforts to 'liberalise' public attitudes. The unenlightened populace might succumb to a 'moral panic' which increases their latent 'homophobia'."

He then proceeds to dismiss the efforts of moral panic theorists to turn attention to the ways in which the media construct particular kinds of events, such as "mugging" in the 1970s, showing that street violence is by no means a modern phenomenon, and that its victims are in fact mostly blacks and Asians – members of the very groups which the press "blames" for muggings in the first place. He is particularly critical and disparaging of groups like the London Gay Teenage Group, and seems extremely upset at the exposure of "heterosexism in the school curriculum", though he displaces his own impatience with such attitudes back on to the sociologists who have studied them.

Irony is heaped on irony in order to belittle medical and sociological supporters of gay teenagers and gay identity as such. His aim is to show evidence of a deafening chorus of encouragement for the situation of lesbians and gay men in contemporary Britain.

> "In fact," he concludes, "there has not been a moral panic about Aids – headlines of course, but only sociologists take headlines that seriously ... What there have been are various attempts by political activists, academics and assorted unappointed spokespersons for 'the gay community' to politicise homosexuality, relativise moral standards, make homosexuality not only tolerated but regarded as just as normal as heterosexuality, to remove obstacles to it and thus, inevitably, extend the incidence of homosexual practice."

This is the nub of the matter. Like the author of the 1960s sex education handbook quoted earlier, Anderson clearly dreads what he regards as the possible "extension" of homosexuality. He dreads the actual sexual diversity of his own readership, which he addresses in a compact of presumed collective heterosexual scorn for positively identified gay men. He can cope "at a personal level" with "homosexuals among my friends"; what he recognises is precisely the distance between the cowed subservient identity of the "homosexual" and the scandalously affirmative presence of the gay man.

> "Should not those within Judaism, and Christian churches, Islam and among half-churched but traditionally inclined parents, and the many homosexuals who do not approve of homosexual proselytisation, start to be concerned? In short, what we need is a little *more* moral panic?"

So the piece moves full circle, from a blanket dismissal of those who have drawn attention to the problems of contemporary Aids commentary, to a blanket injunction against gay culture. Aids does not concern him in the least, save as a platform from which to launch an anti-gay invective.

Whilst Buckley's calls for tattooing and "more drastic segregation measures" are based on totally spurious and dishonest notions of risk from infection by casual contact, which *The New York Times* had itself dismissed earlier in the year,[18] Anderson's moralising speaks from an older position which stands against sexual diversity as such, in the name of "relativism". Both voices lock together in the knowingly world-weary tone affected by those who feel it their painful but necessary duty to enforce "standards" which should – in their vision of a "decent" society – be beyond debate. But the sheer range of such voices, the accents with which they speak, and the institutions from which they proceed should alert us to the danger of immediately rushing to qualify them all as "homophobic". The concept of phobia derives from the image of Phobos, a Greek deity painted on masks and shields in order to frighten away one's enemies. In clinical terms, it is used to describe attitudes and behaviour which enable invididuals to *avoid* what they are frightened by. Phobias are essentially defensive mechanisms, whereby the unconscious projects out onto some object or class of objects anxieties which are in fact internal and instinctual. This presents obvious problems for most of the phenomena commonly characterised as "homophobic", since far from avoiding a taboo and terrifying object, they appear to rush to confront it directly.

The notion of homophobia was initially conceived in the United States in the immediate wake of Gay Liberation, as both a disease and an attitude "held by many non-homosexuals and perhaps by the majority of homosexuals in countries where there is discrimination against homosexuals."[19] It thus has to describe both homosexual and heterosexual attitudes towards homosexuality. In effect, the term merely reversed the widespread tendency to pathologise all forms of homosexual desire and acts as symptoms of a single underlying "perversion", whilst accepting and reinforcing the authority of medical, psychiatric and legal institutions to define "the perverse". It remains most unlikely that we shall find a single "cause" which might explain the entire range of hostile responses to homosexuality, any more than we might find such a single "cause" for the entire range of homosexual desire itself. Ironically, the discourse of "homophobia" turns out to be as reductive as the explanations of homosexuality which it ostensibly seeks to counter.

Unsurprisingly, the spectrum of attitudes towards homosexuality is informed by attitudes towards sexuality as a whole, which are dictated and directed by much larger and more complex historical issues than the concept of phobia can address on its own. This is not, however, to conclude that we can simply collapse together social and psychic factors as if these were subject to the same determining forces. Thus, however similar they may appear, we should not identify the specific local cultural framing of homosexuality, with individual psychic responses, as if they were aspects of the same phenomenon. Otherwise we will merely confuse conscious hostility to homo-sexuality, which is rooted in religious, moral or political codes and values, with other forms of unconscious displaced misogyny, gender anxiety and, on occasion, repressed homosexual desire turning back compulsively against its own forbidden object.

To begin with, we may fairly detect specific "structures of feeling" in both Britain and the United States over the presence of homosexuality in both cultures. Historically, concern has been focused on individual sexual acts, proscribed in law and theology. Thus, in Britain public torture and executions for sodomy persisted well into the nineteenth century, in ways which had not been equalled elsewhere in Europe for more than 200 years.[20] Public attitudes towards homosexuality evidently sustained a xenophobic cultural tradition which had, in the Reformation period, redirected the traditional Roman Catholic persecution of heretics towards Roman Catholics themselves, seen as agents of hostile foreign powers. The sheer scale of the persecution of homosexuals in Britain suggests that this virulent strain of British nationalism found a new focus in the course of the seventeenth century on those who could similarly be identified as "enemies within", threats to the unity of a political dominion which was in any case unstable. The unity of the United

Kingdom has, after all, always resulted from the economic exploitation and political domination by the English of their confederated neighbours: the Scots, Welsh and Irish. Thus the prosecution of the "sodomite" was one aspect of an intensely aggressive nationalism which turned an equally ferocious attention to gypsies, witches, Christian sectarians, Jews and other social groups whose styles of life remained distinct from their host society. The significance of the relations between racism and anti-homosexual attitudes amongst the "respectable" middle classes of England and other modern Western nation states right up to the present day remains in urgent need of explanation by cultural historians. It is, however, safe to conclude that the structures of modern national identity, as they are lived out in the course of everyday life, remain massively dependent on an ideological framework which is able at any point to draw instant analogies between the individual family unit and the nation, understood as a familial entity. In this context we might consider the role of the Royal Family in Britain, which provides both a glamorous "human" face for abstract national identity, and an ideal and supposedly timeless object for emulation for individual subjects. The image of the American Presidential family plays a similar role in the United States, appearing as both the face of government and at the same time an ordinary family, supposedly very much like any other.

That lesbians and gay men are still so universally excluded from ordinary cultural pictures of family life does not help the process of identifying us as national subjects, whether British or American. This in turn can lead to frightening consequences in relation to the treatment of people with Aids, as implied in a recent interview with the Scottish Health Minister, John MacKay, who argued against the distribution of disposable syringes to drug users, which would make needle sharing impossible, on the grounds "that heroin addiction is wrong, and that we ought not as a government – as a country – be encouraging it by giving people the means".[21] That people do not appear to have any difficulty in obtaining needles without government support seems not to have occurred to him, nor that IV drug-users are as fully citizens of the UK as anybody else, and in need of particular help at this time. Blaming the spread of Aids on gay men, he commented that,

> "we are going to be asked to spend a lot of money on a disease which could easily be prevented by people changing their lifestyles... I think this is a straightforward moral issue."

Were there a cholera outbreak in Glasgow he would doubtless show the same "common sense" by recommending local residents to give up the filthy habit of drinking water. Similar attitudes are rife in the United States where, for example, the Reverend Enrique Rueda (who courageously "posed" as a gay man during his researches) has written of homosexuality as a "reservoir of disease", and gay couples as "a form of cancer", whilst concluding that the "homosexual community could be considered a diseased portion of the body politic".[22]

Such opinions clearly denote the active legacy of moral and theological debates which entirely pre-date the modern period, yet which remain available to make sense of any aspect of contemporary life in a far from fossilised discourse of disease and contagion. We should recall that the very notion of "the homosexual" as a distinct type of person, defined primarily in relation to particular sexual acts, emerged in the last century at the interstices of a host of overlapping discourses concerning sickness, contamination and genetic throw-backs, and was regarded as the most concrete evidence of the results of indecency, depravity and uncleanliness. The category of "the homosexual" personified such concerns, revealing an unhealthy sexual appetite in an unhealthy body, doubly threatening because not so readily identifiable as other agents of filth and degradation – prostitutes, the poor, the mad, blacks, the physical and moral delinquents of every slum in Europe and America. Hence the implication, so clearly evident throughout Aids commentary, that the modern gay man belongs to a particular order of felony – that of the wanton, deliberately self-degrading and disgusting degenerate. To describe such attitudes as "phobic" is, in a sense, to lend them a spurious psychological dignity which they do not deserve. The situation of those who suffer from clinical phobias is generally extremely unpleasant and debilitating, and beyond their conscious control. What we hear in the garbage spewed forth by men like MacKay is mere bigotry, however interesting it may be to future historians of late twentieth-century moral and sexual hypocrisy.

Such attitudes should be distinguished from those motivated by gender anxieties, which are an inevitable by-product of the psychic violence involved in the processes which attempt to homogenise all children towards the fixed identities of adult heterosexuality. It is easy to detect a variety of specific defences against what are understood as "passive" sexual acts, on the part of men whose sense of self is constructed around notions of sexual "activity".[23] Such obsessions result from attempts to resolve psychic conflicts due to ambivalence, in which one contending emotion or wish is inflated whilst the other vanishes. The result is what Freud calls a "reaction-formation",[24] which is frequently rigid and compulsive, and in relation to explicit hostility towards homosexuality, often leads directly to results quite opposite to those consciously intended. This is the situation of "queer bashers", whose actual violence often leads to a suspicion of connection with the objects of their exaggeratedly hostile behaviour. As Laplanche and Pontalis have argued, "does not the housewife who is obsessed with cleanliness end up by concentrating her whole existence on dust and dirt?".[25] We must, however, distinguish between such obsessional behaviour, which may become pathological to the extent of taking over an entire personality, and strictly phobic behaviour, where, as Freud points out,

> "the ego behaves as if the danger of a development of anxiety threatened it not from the direction of an instinctual impulse but from the direction of a perception, and it is thus enabled to react against this external danger with the attempts at flight represented by phobic avoidances".[26]

In this respect it seems likely that cases of extreme verbal or physical violence towards lesbians and gay men and, by extension, the whole topic of Aids, result either from reaction-formations developed to defend the individual against some repressed emotion or wish within him or herself, or else from other displaced and strictly speaking phobic anxieties projected on to gay men, about gender, sexual potency or even career prospects. In some cases, as I have suggested, this may be symptomatic of displaced mysogyny, with a hatred of what is projected as "passive" and therefore female, sanctioned by the subject's dominant heterosexual drives. In other cases an overriding sense of shame concerning excretory functions may be projected onto men (or women) whose sexuality seems to expose and even celebrate the object of disgust which, Freud reminds us, always also bears the imprint of desire.

Here we should stop to consider one particular aspect of Aids commentary which clearly intersects with obsessional attitudes towards homosexuality, namely the tendency to attribute Aids intrinsically to sodomy, and thence to the domain of the "unnatural". Anal sex, especially between men, causes widespread anxiety among many different people, including an American born again Christian follower of Anita Bryant, who counsels gay men against homosexuality on the grounds that the appropriate sexual parts do not "fit" between members of the same sex – a penis does not supposedly "fit" a mouth or a rectum (male or female in both cases).[27] Another influential moral majority spokesman in America claims that if the Centers for Disease Control "would just come out and make a list of what homosexuals do, I think the public debate would essentially be over in a week", referring to calls for mass quarantining. He confidently assumes a shared public "disgust" equal to his own, which is, I suspect, typical self-deception on the part of neo-conservative, born again and moral majority campaigners alike. Criticising Dr James Mason, the Acting Assistant Secretary of Health and Human Sciences at the CDC, who had commented that he saw no difference between monogamous homosexuality and monogamous heterosexuality, he exclaims:

> "Now, there's obviously something wrong with his bio- · logical training ... the idea that a vagina is the same as a rectum, or vice versa ... If homosexuals didn't drink urine, ingest faeces, and practise rectal intercourse and swallow faeces, probably [here he gave a big laugh] they wouldn't get very many diseases."[28]

This man's imagination runs riot to the most extreme and bizarre aspects of human sexual behaviour in much the same way that other writers rush towards the most obscure and wildly extreme possibilities of HIV transmission. Paul Morrissey, for example, snatched away a Gay Pride poster at a public gay community meeting with the Mayor of New York, shouting "Shame, shame, shame", having claimed at a previous meeting about the New York gay rights bill that people were intentionally sneezing on him in order to give him Aids.[29] The endlessly repeated medical information that the HIV virus cannot be contracted like tuberculosis or smallpox via air-borne droplets clearly has no persuasive effect whatsoever on such states of mind.

In such cases a multiple disturbance is evidently taking place, involving symbolic social and psychic codes about the supposedly "correct" and "natural" uses of the body and, by extension, the entire social order. This degree of obsessive language and behaviour is inseparable from a particular type of sexual identity, regardless of its own object-choice, which can only consciously accept sex as the insertion of a penis into a vagina, within marriage, and preferably for the sole purpose of procreation. This kind of neurosis always involves a certain prosecution of the self, providing a clean moral and physical bill of health, a sense of privilege, solidarity, superiority and cleanliness which is significantly like the type of Nazi anti-semitism and homophobia that drew on similar anxieties about the dirty, the perverse and the degenerate.

In this context we should also place the writings of populist sociobiologists like Glenn Wilson, whom I take to stand for a wide and influential school of sexual commentators, and who does not remain silent on the subject of homosexuality.[30] Lesbians and gay men are of particular interest to the "evolutionary theorist", he explains, because we supposedly exhibit "pure" sexual and gender characteristics, having no need "to compromise with the differing proclivities of the opposite sex". In this version of the world, gay men supposedly inhabit some kind of no-woman's land, completely untouched by, and unconscious of, the opposite sex. Dismissed on the one hand as "failed" heterosexuals, we are restored on the other as ideal demonstrations of unadulterated masculine and feminine sex-drives. Nor is he short on explanations of homosexuality, which apparently range from brain lesions to forceps delivery and infantile meningitis. You can take your pick. His own preferred theory is that when Mother Nature doles out "competitive", "aggressive" masculinity, some men "miss out" and find it "comfortable and convenient to assume certain aspects of the female role ... Others, feeling a need for some kind of substitute, might find it easier to make contact with these submissive males rather than compete against the top men for the females". Thus "reproducing is left to those males with the most vigour and strength to contribute to the species". This staggering flight of sociobiological fancy is, he concedes, "rather insulting to homosexuals". But at least he does allow us some place at the foot of the evolutionary tree to be socially "useful", as artists and philosophers... Unfortunately, some aspects of this farrago of nonsense are echoed by some feminists, in particular the vision of gay men as somehow embodying "manliness" at its purest and most extreme, as in the work of Andrea Dworkin, for whom we represent the very apogee of patriarchal iniquity.[31] But with Wilson we are back in the familiar world of homophobic science, where all gay men must be either "active" or "passive" because, apparently, that is the case for men and women. Here we are, in any case, already ideologically and psychologically down-wind of Belsen, when we read gruesome reports of "compulsive sexual deviations that have been surgically removed along with a focal epilepsy".[32]

Whatever variant the "lock-and-key" explanation of human sexuality takes up, it always fails to recognise the fundamental diversity of sexual choice and behaviour, and the multivalence of all our body parts. As one commentator has observed, "sex is sexy because it's more than natural selection. It's sex."[33] Thus we may return to the American attorney involved in the failed attempt to challenge the state of Georgia's anti-sodomy statutes, who argued that the state cannot legislate "a catalogue of what body parts can touch".[34] This, however, is precisely the intention which lay behind the recent attempt by a prominent right-wing British politician to introduce new legislation controlling the exhibition of sex on television – if

> "it depicts visually, and in actual or simulated form, acts of masturbation, sodomy, oral/genital connection, the lewd exhibition of genital organs or excretory functions, cannibalism, bestiality, mutilation or vicious cruelty towards persons or animals".[35]

Whether they emanate from neo-conservatism, Christian fundamentalism, sociobiology or feminism, all these positions share a common aim to ground a narrow, normative theory of human nature in biology. Recalling the misery and anguish – and physical danger – which homophobia leads to for lesbians and gay men, we need to be far more sensitive to the assumptions our society makes about the supposed "nature" of the natural world, and what analogies are held to be relevant between human beings and members of other species. In this respect we can identify the whole of medical education as it trains doctors and nurses and affects their career prospects, as one major vector of homophobic science, together with all the other academic disciplines – criminology, social psychology, politics, and so on – which possess the power to institutionalise and disseminate evaluative sexual definitions and discourses. It is in this manner that obsessional neuroses and phobias towards homosexuality are constantly negotiating with the larger cultural and historical social forces that are always ready and waiting, fully armed and mobilised against homosexual desire.

We may thus begin to account for the *systematic misinformation* which is so widespread throughout Aids commentary, as we have already seen. It is also in this context that we must seriously consider the forceful argument of Dr Joseph Sonnabend that

> "the rectum is a sexual organ, and it deserves the respect that a penis gets and a vagina gets. Anal intercourse is a central sexual activity, and it should be supported ... Everybody's too embarrassed to even contemplate this ... In fact, it's terribly important to actually do this, because anal intercourse has been the central activity for gay men and for some women for all of history. It's not going to go away because it's been declared unhealthy and unsound at this moment. It's become unhealthy ... It's not the act itself, but the fact that it becomes a vehicle for infection ... That's an unfortunate hazard. What I'm trying to say is that we have to recognise what is hazardous, but at the same time, we shouldn't undermine an act that's important to celebrate,

> just because it's under attack by the straight community.
> And this attack should not be joined by gay men."[36]

This is not merely another reverse discourse, but offers a fundamental opportunity to re-think and re-evaluate our entire approach towards the human body and questions of sexual pleasure and identity. It also offers an important strategy of resistance to media commentators like the comedian Eddie Murphy, now notorious for his Aids jokes, who solemnly described to *Rolling Stone* in 1984 how,

> "faggots... have nothing to fucking do but sit around with tight asses and feel like people are pointing at them... The way I feel about it is, what they did helped my album because the majority of the country is heterosexual, and they read that homosexuals don't like Eddie Murphy and they think, 'hey, all right'..."

We must actively support organisations such as the national Campaign for Press and Broadcasting Freedom in Britain, and comparable American institutions, to ensure that the finger felt to be pointing is ours. At the 1985 annual Gay and Lesbian Freedom parade in Columbus, Ohio, anti-gay protestors even hired a light aircraft to circumnavigate the day's proceedings trailing a banner which read "AIDS – God's curse on Homos". We have to be equally enterprising, to force our presence and our values on institutions which have hitherto felt confident enough to negate our very existence. We have to campaign and organise in order to enter the amphitheatre of Aids commentary effectively and unapologetically on our own terms. This is particularly important, since Aids commentary is also "news", and becomes internationally syndicated, "taking off" from its local origins into a much larger trans-Atlantic currency.

Thus, on the 8.00 news on BBC Radio Four one morning recently, I listened to a Dr Adrian Rogers, who had written to a medical journal calling for the "removal" of "Aids victims" to quarantine centres because, as he put it, "hundreds of people are going to die".[37] Needless to say he was not referring to gay men, as was made clear from his warning about "moral behaviour", claiming, against all the available evidence, that there is no evidence of changes in sexual behaviour. This kind of implicit ideological slippage from "homosexuality" to "promiscuity" to Aids is a commonplace of far too much Aids commentary. In the case of Dr Rogers, and so many like him, an overtly "moral" discourse articulates a social *and* psychological inability to accept that morality is not singular and universal, but a site of conflicting definitions and interests. In a similar vein Paul

Cameron, an American consultant to Republican representative William Dannemeyer, has described his concern that "this whole epidemic is being significantly mishandled ... had a quarantine been imposed in '81 we probably would be looking at a very small expenditure". Expenditure of what, one might immediately ask, especially in the United States, which so conspicuously lacks anything remotely resembling an adequate public health programme. Medical profiteering from Aids in the home of "free enterprise" remains one of the single most nauseating aspects of the entire epidemic. I should, however, add that on a recent visit to Dallas I found that gay men in a community already devastated by Aids did not by any means agree on the need for a Medicare programme along the lines of the British National Health Service. However clearly the threat of Aids demonstrates that the one thing all human beings have in common is the fact of our common mortality, this does not automatically over-ride other political and ideological considerations of economic profitability, the "threat" of creeping communism, and so on.

It should be noted that Dr Rogers speaks on behalf of the far right Conservative Family Campaign, which was a major force behind the recent revision of the Education Act which took control of sex education out of the hands of teachers. Their intentions were clearly stated in *The Times* of 23 September, 1986:

> "to save a generation from the immoral propaganda for promiscuity, homosexuality, anti-marriage views, fornication, and encouragement of children to experiment with sex, which has passed in far too many schools during the last two decades as health education".

As a result, parents may refuse to allow their children to attend classes concerning Aids or Safer Sex information, whilst individual headteachers can forbid sex education in its entirety from the curriculum of their schools. Hence Britain currently faces an extraordinary situation in which the Government attempts to educate the population about Aids through a massive national information campaign, whilst remaining steadfastly opposed to sex education in schools. In this context we should note that according to national figures published in the *Guardian* on 3 March, 1987, only 3.9 per cent of 649 women having abortions had even discussed condoms with their teachers. One of the major problems facing those involved in Aids information work in the coming years thus concerns not so much individual government policies, as conflicts and contradictions between different policies, and different ministerial departments. Many young people will die of Aids in Britain as the *direct* result of the lobbying power of the Conservative Family Campaign and kindred organisations of the lunatic right, whose "morality" evidently prefers the spectacle of dead children to the reform of our appalling national sexual ignorance – an ignorance which is scrupulously maintained with the full force of law.

Fortunately, the same BBC news broadcast "balanced" the rantings of Dr Rogers with the saner voice of Dr Peter Jones from Newcastle, who pointed out that with an estimate of some five to fifteen million people infected by the HIV virus, according to the World Health Organisation, notions of quarantine appear somewhat ridiculous. All that is needed in the care of actual people with Aids is ordinary medical hygiene, he added, calling for people like Dr Rogers to come down from their moral pedestals and think for a moment what it is like to be infected. People with Aids, he insisted, need "to be loved, held and cherished". That is certainly the voice of sanity, but it is rarely heard above the general din of prejudice, hatred, obsession and phobia.

It is still probably more helpful than not to retain the notion of "homophobia", at least as a collective term referring to the whole range of negative evaluations of homosexuality *per se*, as long as this does not lead us to assume a single underlying and all-determining factor at work behind every example of irrational anti-gay prejudice. It is especially important for lesbians and gay men not to collapse social and psychic issues together, since this is what is so frequently done to us, either pathologising our entire culture in all its diversity as the product of neurosis, or suggesting that homosexual desire is merely learned, and therefore curable by enforced unlearning. That no such suggestions have ever been made about heterosexuality, except by the lunatic fringe of the women's movement,[38] remains, however, enormously significant. The full depth, extent, variety and virulence of homophobia in Western society passes all but unnoticed in all the major disciplines which purport to explain its social and psychic structures – sociology, anthropology, linguistics, history, cultural studies, medicine and psychoanalysis alike. All these disciplines share a normative, taken-for-granted assumption that the central cultural and social subject of their enquiries is exclusively heterosexual. This involves a degree of presumably defensive disavowal unparalleled in contemporary thought. And it is a disavowal which spills out into all the leading institutions which direct and govern our lives. We should not do this society the service of retreating into isolationist fantasies about the possibility of our own complete autonomy, when such fantasies merely echo, in reverse, the dominant attitudes and wishes of a vicious, ignorant and hypocritically concupiscent social order, with which we are obliged –

now more than ever – to contend. This is nowhere more pressingly the case than in relation to laws defining obscenity and indecency, which already clamp menacingly around lesbian and gay culture in all its forms, including the distribution of information about Safer Sex – at this moment in time our only protection against the ravages of Aids.

Chapter Four

Aids, pornography and law

In all its variant forms, modern sexuality is policed by laws which regulate and oversee sexual desires, actions and identities. Laws determine child custody rights, ages of sexual consent (currently fixed in Great Britain as sixteen for heterosexual and twenty-one for homosexual acts), immigration, and the very distinction between male and female. However, as Paul Hirst has recently written,

> "the law is not an entity, it is a very complex set of rules and institutions, persons and activities, and it is by no means consistent in its action. There is no legal instance specifying the attributes of persons consistently and coherently".[1]

This point is extremely important to bear in mind as we move to consider the ways in which different laws operate to interrupt or forbid the circulation of images and texts concerning both homosexuality and information about Aids. Whilst the law has not set out in either Britain or America deliberately to proscribe discussion of Aids, that in effect has been the case, given the closure of "adult" bookstores in the name of indecency laws in both countries, and as a result of Customs and Excise interventions in Britain. Thus, for example, a hapless tourist returning to the UK had a copy of the national American gay newspaper *The Advocate* seized at London's Gatwick airport, together with a video tape, a *Colt* calendar, and some twenty sex magazines. This, in spite of a directive issued to customs officers in June, 1978, which clearly states that, with the significant exception of child pornography, they are not permitted to detain small quantities of obscene or indecent books or magazines when they are intended solely for the personal use of an incoming traveller.[2]

Any gay man returning to Britain from the United States in recent years would want to bring copies of *The Advocate* and *New York Native* with him, since they contain the only sustained information and debates concerning the Aids epidemic, and have been effectively illegal in this country since British Customs' 1984 "Operation Tiger" against London's Gay's The Word bookshop, the second largest lesbian and gay community bookstore in the world. Following raids on the shop itself, and the homes of three of its directors, Customs and Excise adopted two lines of attack. The first concerned a total of one hundred criminal charges against the eight directors, shop manager Paul Hegarty, and Gay's The Word as a private limited company. The second involved the seizure of 142 imported titles on the grounds that they were "indecent" or "obscene", a distinction which I shall come on to discuss in greater detail. Prosecutions proceeded from the Customs Consolidation Act of 1876, which does not establish specific criteria differentiating obscenity from in-decency, and is concerned solely with what the "ordinary man in the street" might consider to be in "poor taste". Needless to say, the imaginary man-in-the-street is constructed as exclusively hetero-sexual and, in this instance, virulently homophobic. The Gay's The Word case, to which I will return, should also be regarded in the larger context of raids and prosecutions of shops and clubs selling gay magazines and periodicals which take place with grim and monotonous regularity throughout the United Kingdom. Thus, in October, 1985, North London magistrates were able to fine the publishers of Britain's only nationally distributed gay newspaper, *Gay Times*, over £5,000 for sending out "indecent materials" through the post. That these "materials" contained no explicit sex scenes, only male nudes, and were being sent to paying subscribers, mattered not one jot. At another extreme of this current of legislative attention we should also locate the recently failed Churchill Amendment Bill in Britain, which would have effectively criminalised all images of homosexuality within British culture.

What was radically new about the proposed amendment was its extension of previous legal definitions of obscenity beyond existing principles of harm and offence, to a legal moralism which understands certain categories of subject-matter to be *intrinsically* obscene. This is also the strategy at work in the United States behind the referendum-based campaigns organised in the name of feminism by Andrea Dworkin and Catherine MacKinnon, which would bring the term "pornography" into legal discourses for the first time as a self-evident category.[3] This would also seem to be the aim of the American Attorney General's recent Commission on Pornography, which endorses and solicits prosecutions by individuals of materials which lie far beyond the province of existing American obscenity laws, including anything that "some citizens may find dangerous or offensive or immoral".[4] All these positions share a common determination to iron out all inconsistencies and complexities within current legislations surrounding sexuality, and to replace them with fixed codes regulating the production, distribution and consumption of all sexual materials according to strict universalising content-based definitions of "pornography". It is thus the ambition of this strategy to wrench away all questions of morality from the protective claims of "privacy", as encoded in prèsent legislations, and to force them into the public domain. The strategy regards pornography, defined in terms which are not open to question, as *intrinsically* harmful. In this manner the morality of one particular lobby group would be legally binding across an entire society in such a way that sexual diversity, and many forms of political and cultural diversity, would become effectively criminalised.

Such an approach is radically inconsistent with previous post-war legal attitudes towards the relations between legislation and sexual conduct, which Beverley Brown has summarised as the "Wolfenden Strategy", after the influential Wolfenden Report of 1957, which led eventually to the partial decriminalisation of homosexuality in Britain in the Sexual Offences Act of 1967. Wolfenden Strategy was intended to establish a firm distinction between the domains of the public and private, involving "a shrinking of legislative control over personal conduct combined with a more rigorous policing of the cordon representing the public domain".[5] Thus, in the words of Jeffrey Weeks, "the duty of law is to regulate public order and to maintain acceptable (though by implication changing) standards of public decency, not to patrol personal life".[6] The result, as he points out, has been confusion

> "over the definition of 'private' (especially with regard to homosexuality and pornography, where the definition constantly seems to shift) and over 'consent', which is crucial to the liberal approach".[7]

Whilst American law is always ultimately gauged against the Constitution and Bill of Rights, in Britain liberalism is *sui generis*, and open to much wider interpretations and variations of effect. It is precisely this legal latitude which the new legal moralism intends to eradicate once and for all.

Whilst I do not wish to collapse British and American law into a semblance of spurious unity, I think we can distinguish a set of shared issues. Whilst ostensibly defending the rights of "consenting adults in public", Wolfenden Strategy led to a widespread displacement of sexual attention away from the home, in the larger direction of "public" places, which were henceforth to be rigorously – and at times obsessively – policed. This has involved an intensive degree of moral management on the part of the police force, as well as welfare agencies, criminologists, sociologists of "deviance", professional psychologists, journalists and so on. The result is low level but permanent regulation, ceaselessly scrutinising the entire fabric of social life for tell-tale signs of "dangerous" sexualities. In this way homosexuality has become reframed as a "problem" of public life rather than personal identity, at the same time fuelling and reinforcing older notions of risk to the (heterosexual) community at large. So, whereas Wolfenden Strategy tried to protect what were regarded as especially vulnerable groups, particularly children, what we may now tentatively identify as Post Wolfenden Strategy seeks instead to establish a principle of *universal* vulnerability. Universal, that is, except for the would-be legislators of the new right, who, strapped safely to the mast of moral absolutism, remain severely immune to our siren charms. Thus, whether or not we live in states or countries where homosexuality is still a criminal offence, a legal gaze invariably surveys our lives, together with the marginally less obtrusive attentions of other agencies of moral regulation, from social workers to the local Neighbourhood Watch scheme. Our lives are constantly the subject of fascinated disapproval, in our homes and on the streets, and are lived out in relation to powerful institutions which we rarely feel brushing past us in the course of everyday life, but nonetheless know are there.

We thus face two distinct sets of problems, firstly concerning the actual workings of Wolfenden Strategy and, secondly, concerning the still more threatening implications of Post-Wolfenden Strategy. In effect we are being invited to choose whether we prefer to regard homosexuality as indecent and/or obscene, or intrinsically "pornographic". It is this paradox which I want now to explore, emphasising that our understanding of the issues involved in this particular debate are of pressing and immediate significance to our everyday lives, regardless of our sexuality. What is at stake is no less than the existence of sexual debate and sexual politics. To begin with we need to grasp the significance of current, operative legislation.

In the United States "obscenity" is a legal term defined by the Supreme Court through the application of a "three-pronged test": if (a) the average person, applying contemporary community standards, finds that a work as a whole appeals to prurient interests and (b) the work depicts and describes in a "patently offensive way" sexual conduct, and (c) it lacks serious literary, artistic, political or scientific value, it is obscene.[8] As Donna Turley explains, "criminal obscenity statutes depend on the state to prosecute and generally provide for financial and penal sanctions and for the censoring of those materials". The goal of the Meese Commission and of local referendum-based feminist campaigners like Andrea Dworkin is to enable anyone to bring a civil suit against anything deemed to be "offensive" and hence "pornographic", with no grounds for appeal or exclusion clauses as in the present obscenity law. This is why the alignment of feminists and party politicians of the left and right alike is so ominous, since it enables the legal moralist to couch his or her case in the name of women's rights. Anything that any individual woman construed as offensive could be prosecuted as an aspect of the subordination of all women. As Turley continues,

"implicit in the arguments of the anti-pornography campaign is the assumption that there exists a female sexuality that is excluded from most pornography and sex... romantic, egalitarian, natural, gentle, free of power dynamics, monogamous, emotional, nurturing and spontaneous. This feminist prescription reflects and reproduces the dominant cultural assumptions about women, [and is premised] on the notion that women are victims of sex and that sex is degrading to women but not to men".[9]

This position clearly inherits from the general absence in nineteenth-century thought of "any concept of female sexuality which is independent of men's",[10] and derives its political vision from Victorian morality, which Weeks presents as organised through a series

"of ideological separations: between family and society, between the restraint of the domestic circle and the temptations of promiscuity; between the privacy, leisure and comforts of the home and the tensions and competitiveness of work".[11]

Hence the emergence of a monolithic moralism organised around the family unit, which remains as central a rallying point for many of today's feminists and neo-conservatives, as it was for earlier generations of social purity campaigners in both traditions.

The irony of this tactical alliance has been neatly summarised by Richard Summerhill, who explores the distinction between feminist criticisms of pornography on the grounds that it degrades women, and right wing criticisms that it is itself intrinsically degrading. Thus,

"in much of current feminist thought, pornography is looked upon as a symptom of *excessive* control by patriarchal males... To conservatives, porn represents a completely unrelated set of problems... Porn, like prostitution and homosexuality, weakens... by turning people's sexual interests away from social benefit (babies and self-control for its own sake) and towards self-indulgence and self-gratification. In other words, porn contains a threat of *insufficient* control... This is the porn that 'is degrading', the passive form of pornographic menace. It causes people to break down from within as if they were diseased, and it rots out the mortar joining the bricks of the social structure. Porn seems a form of degradation which is insidious and 'filthy' in nature: quite unlike the active, grinding, nasty sort of degradation visioned by feminists".[12]

It is just this slippage from notions of passive menace to the menace of male sexual passivity which activates the alignment of pornography to Aids which I have already described. As an American commentator writes:

"The opponents of pornography, from fundamentalists to radical feminists, are in agreement: pornography is 'sick'. Not bad, boring, silly, useless... Porn is described as an 'epidemic' in the same way that Aids has. The pornographer is seen as a vampire: he wishes to 'infect' society and must be wiped out... Jerry Falwell inveighs against smut as if it's a sub-genre of 'sick' homosexuality; for Robin Morgan, 'pornography is the theory, and rape the practice... Pornography can't be 'sick' because sexuality isn't 'sick'. The pornographic 'sickness' doesn't reside in the works of pornography, but in the minds of erotophobes... Attacking porn for contributing to the number of Aids cases betrays a fundamental misunderstanding of both porn and disease. A disease has no conscience. Being 'good' – for example – will not prevent you from getting sick".[13]

The tragedy nonetheless remains that so many feminists seem unable to recognise that the power of the hands into which they are playing far exceeds the remotest possibilities of harm caused by explicit sexual materials. However, as Chris Bearchell writes, although

"the power of a critique of fundamental social structures is lost as individual men are seen as the source of women's problems... there are still feminists who have the important targets in sight... They know that an obsession with victimhood can derail a movement that must concern itself with power – who has it, how they got it, and how to take it for ourselves. It must be up to those feminists to point out the ever-more-apparent dangers of allegiances with those who, despite their superficial commitment to common concerns, are enemies of freedom and justice".[14]

In Britain the situation is still more complex, given the existence of distinct notions of both indecency and obscenity in Common and Statute law. So, whilst there is no conception of "pornography" as such in British jurisprudence, it is clear that the formulation of laws concerning concepts of obscenity and indecency are enacted in the name of national and community standards which are exclusively heterosexual. Such laws systematically equate the "national subject" with the "average person" as the locus of moral judgement and at the same time of potential vulnerability. Indeed, the entire Wolfenden Strategy may be read as a complex discourse on the subject of sexual vulnerability, anxiously protecting those held to be at special risk from potential "corruption". Thus a normative yet somehow ever-threatened heterosexuality is inscribed at the heart of the institution of law.

In this context we might contrast the relative national identities involved in being American or British. American-ness operates as a federal identity, working to lock together a complex of more intimate, variable identifications – regional, racial, religious, political and so on. Thus the black liberal Texan gay Baptist is no less "American" than a lesbian WASP from California, or a New York Jewish democrat mother of five. British-ness, on the contrary, is a subject-identity unified in relation to parliament and the monarchy, rather than to the democratic ideal of a constitution. Just as England hegemonises the rest of the UK in political authority, so Britishness emerges as an *initial* term, rather than a result, possessing a strong power of precedence over and above regional, racial, economic, political and other differences. In a history of the symbols of national identity, the Restoration of the Monarchy would rank beside the American Declaration of Independence. Thus it is that gay politics have been far more successful in America, where a powerful tradition of civil rights consciousness preceded the emergence of the gay movement, which has established the presence of lesbians and gay men as a fundamental category within the larger social formation, by analogy with the other identities of race, religion, national origin and so on. This has not been the case in England, where there was no such powerful civil rights model, and where gay political energies were more frequently channelled into a far left politics which was far more interested in recruiting statistics into Party membership, than in actual sexual politics. So Britain has still not seen even a primitive equivalent to the widespread civil rights awareness which so informs American lesbian and gay culture, except under the vulnerable left wing of the Labour Party, as it ran London under the late and extremely lamented Greater London Council. Class politics remain as tragically incompatible as ever with libertarian politics in the UK.

In the absence of a written British constitution, it remains impossible to defend lesbian and gay culture in any of its forms against arbitrary prosecution according to the whim of local Customs officials, Post Office agents, or police superintendants. There is no national equivalent to the First Amendment to the American Constitution, in the name of which the US Post Office was successfully challenged by the Athletic Model Guild and others in the course of the 1950s, thereby guaranteeing a freedom of distribution for sexual materials which has never existed in Britain.

Paul Crane summarises the situation, distinguishing

> "two types of legal censorship on explicit sexual materials: '(1) the prohibition of "obscene" material likely to "deprave and corrupt" readers or viewers; (2) laws that permit the police to confiscate "indecent" material likely to embarrass the "ordinary citizen".'"[15]

Thus, although as we have seen, the law does not define "pornography", Annette Kuhn points out that

> "one of the effects of legal discourse may well be to construct a body of representations which are subject to regulation by proscription or restriction . . . by appealing to a regulatory discourse which, as such, both precedes and exceeds pornography".[16]

Whilst the indecency laws are endlessly used to intervene in gay culture, with raids on bookshops and so on, the Obscene Publications Act of 1959 is much less frequently put into action. As Annette Kuhn again observes:

> "the legal test of obscenity is extremely stringent: not only must a tendency to deprave and corrupt be established in relation to a particular article, which is difficult in itself, but the article must also be taken as a whole, and the whole must be shown to have a deleterious moral effect on those most likely to come into contact with it, as opposed, say, to the population in general, or 'vulnerable' groups such as children or persons leading especially sheltered lives".[17]

Thus the offence of obscenity is concerned with representations in relation to specific social groups who have chosen to be "exposed" to them, whilst the offence of indecency is concerned with the same materials, but from the perspective of those who have not chosen to come into contact with them. Indecency thus involves display, defined in terms of the offence it might cause, rather than moral corruption. Thus a discourse of moral outrage always hovers over legal debates concerning the nature and identity of the audience for pornography, which is simultaneously conceded to want the same materials which might offend other individuals. But for all its fudging of issues concerning the nature of privacy, the Wolfenden Strategy offers considerable latitude for interpretation and defence. It is the recognition of this latitude, and of the extreme difficulty of "successfully" prosecuting obscenity, which has driven Christian and secular fundamentalists alike to more arcane corners of British legal precedence.

It is in this context that we can relate, on the one hand, the resurrection of ancient offences such as Blasphemous Libel, used by the Christian fundamentalist crusader Mary Whitehouse in order to prosecute the now-defunct *Gay News* in 1978 and, on the other, moves like the Churchill Amendment Bill. The recent withdrawal of charges against Gay's The Word bookshop, brought in the name of Customs and Excise law, which fails to distinguish between obscenity and indecency but veers towards the latter, has resulted in an official directive that imported materials should henceforth be judged against existing obscenity legislation. In order to have claimed costs, Gay's The Word would have had to prove either negligence or malice on the part of Customs and Excise, both of which were glaringly obvious in this case, but hard to prove in law. In the event, the contradictions between existing legislations and between British law as a whole and European Economic Community law led to the charges being dropped. In this instance, like many others concerning gay issues, the judicial authority of the EEC has worked against homophobic prosecutions and laws, as in the decision of the European Court of Human Rights in the 1981 Dudgeon *v.* United Kingdom case, which obliged the government to end the total prohibition of homosexuality in private in Northern Ireland. However, by the same token we also find a local residents' association in North London taking their case against a planned lesbian centre in their neighbourhood to the European Court on the grounds that their children would be "threatened" by "unwelcome strangers" in the area. The projection of adult anxieties onto the position of children is entirely congruent with the widespread attitude to family life which regards the home as a place of refuge, entirely beyond regulation, whilst at the same time acknowledging it as a site of fearful dangers, requiring extra-parental policing of many kinds, including the most elaborate legal manoeuvres to guarantee that no child is exposed to anything on television which might bring the slightest blush to adult cheeks.

We can thus expect new initiatives from the self-appointed guardians of public morality over what we should be allowed to read or view, and what we should not. In the Northern Ireland case the government was obliged to call off its hounds and, as gay MP Chris Smith pointed out, "the 1959 Act is by no means perfect, but it's an awful lot better than the open-ended and potentially draconian powers open to Customs at present".[18] It was precisely the Obscene Publications Act which the Churchill Amendment aimed to undermine, by disqualifying any possible defence on behalf of materials deemed potentially obscene for television viewers and others. Significantly, conservative support for the proposed amendment centered on two films made by British gay director Derek Jarman, and the list of subjects which it wished to establish as intrinsically obscene were transparently targeted at homosexuality above all else. This is all the more alarming since its provisions would have obtained anywhere "to which persons under eighteen years of age have access ..." That is, everywhere.

Equally significant, however, was the fact that a mere thirty-one Labour Party MPs voted against the amendment at its second reading, and institutional voices raised focused exclusively on the threat it posed to High Culture – much of Shakespeare would have been immediately unperformable. This is, of course, ludicrous and entirely misses the point that the underlying target was the representation of homosexuality as such. Only one MP pointed out its expressly anti-homosexual purpose, describing it as "obsessively concerned with the anus".[19] The Churchill Amendment affair should remind us of the comparative ease with which homophobic legislation can be introduced on the coat-tails of other Bills, in this case the flurry of legislation concerning the representation of sex, including the Indecent Displays Control Act, 1981; the Local Government (miscellaneous provisions) Act, 1982; the Civil Government (Scotland) Act, 1982; and the Cinematograph Amendment Act of 1982. At the same time, Churchill's Bill was announced as a measure for the protection of children and, as Gayle Rubin observes, "for over a century, no tactic for stirring up erotic hysteria has been as reliable as the appeal to protect children".[20]

Post Wolfenden Strategy is thus deaf to objections from traditional liberal and civil rights positions, since the morality involved is expressly directed against the types of pluralism on behalf of which such objectors plead their cause. The violent lurch to the far right of the American Supreme Court, following the appointment of Reaganite William Rehnquist, also suggests a concerted effort under way to reverse "liberal" precedents of recent decades. It is the function of the Supreme Court to interpret the constitution, in other words the rights of the individual. Whereas it was the Supreme Court which forced Nixon to surrender the Watergate tapes, and championed many civil rights causes, it is now likely to side firmly with what are euphemistically known as "pro-family" positions, in relation to appeals pending over abortion, homosexuality and obscenity charges. The majority decision to rule on behalf of the constitutionality of the state of Georgia's sodomy statute, which makes it illegal for any person to engage in "any sexual act involving the sex organs of one person and the mouth or anus of another" makes clear the legal spirit of the times in America. On 1 July, 1986, the *New York Times* reported that officials from Georgia had decided to proceed with their case after an initial upset, saying "sodomy is an unnatural act and a crime against the laws of God and man. The state also says the law would help reduce the spread of acquired immune deficiency syndrome." Similar laws have been repealed in twenty-six states, while of the twenty-three which still retain them only five apply exclusively to homosexual acts. The states of America are thus extremely disunited in relation to laws surrounding sexuality, and even the tactic of "packing" the Supreme Court does not guarantee immediate, total and uniform power for the New Right. The Georgia decision undoubtedly flew in the face of recent American wisdom, to such an extent that one of the dissenting judges, Harry Blackmun, took the unusual step of reading his opinion to the press that "the right of an individual to conduct intimate relationships in the intimacy of his or her own home seems to me to be the heart of the constitution's protection of privacy".[21]

Debates about the interpretation of "liberty" in relation to notions of "privacy" as an aspect of personal liberty protected by the Fourteenth Amendment are just what the Meese Commission on pornography sets out to avoid in future. Carole S. Vance, who observed the proceedings, describes how,

> "witnesses appearing before the commission were treated in a highly uneven manner. Commissioners accepted virtually any claim made by anti-pornography witnesses as true, asking few probing questions and making only the most cursory requests for evidence or attempts to determine witness credibility. Those who did not support more restriction of sexually explicit speech were often met with rudeness and hostility, and their motives for testifying were impugned".[22]

Recommendations included a "vibrator bill" which would ban as obscene "any device designed or marketed for the stimulation of human genital organs". Here, as in relation to the Georgia sodomy statute decision, Dr Joseph Sonnabend's argument that we should redefine the rectum (and the mouth, I would add) as a sexual organ would produce interesting legal consequences. However, as Vance shrewdly notes that "if these were the McCarthy hearings of sex, they were scripted by *Saturday Night Live* ... The report, and its two volumes, and 1,960 pages, faithfully reflect the censors' fascination with the things they love to hate", listing in alphabetical order "the titles of materials found in sixteen adult bookstores in six cities: 2,370 films, 725 books and 2,325 magazines, beginning with *A Cock Between Friends* and ending with *69 Lesbians Munching*." Anti-pornography slide shows competed with one another to show the most lurid, the most disgusting, the most harmful examples, and

> "witnesses made their unique contributions. Judith Trevillian from Citizens Against Pornography, Michigan, brought a portable tape recorder to reproduce for the audience 'the chilling horror I felt in my kitchen after my first encounter with Dial-a-Porn',"

and a Miami resident described his typically normal, "healthy" childhood, all of which was changed when he came across a deck of hard-core playing cards:

> "By the age of sixteen, after a steady diet of *Playboy*, *Penthouse*, *Scandinavian Children*, etc., I had to see a doctor for neuralgia of the prostate".

After proceeding down the slippery slope still further by having sex with no less than two women, he was saved in the nick of time by divine intervention: "If it weren't for my faith in God and the forgiveness in Jesus Christ, I would now possibly be a pervert, an alcoholic, or dead".[23]

Whilst the overtly "revivalist" tone of such confessions sounds risible in more restrained and secular societies like Britain, we should nonetheless note the core appeal to "family" values which transcends religious witness. Hence we read that the Metropolitan Police Commissioner, Sir Kenneth Newman, apparently identifies

> "a fragmentation of authority as a cause of lower personal standards . . .the breakdown of the family unit was also at the heart of the problem. Fragmentation was also being encouraged by politicians who, 'rather than appeal to the community as a whole, make a policy of appealing to the minorities in it. There have been recent examples of stances taken in order to appeal to sectarian, racial and sexual minorities,' Sir Kenneth said".[24]

He evidently views contemporary Britain within a metaphor of family life, and the law as a uniform, coherent entity to be accepted and respected in its entirety. Further, he pictures the political, racial and sexual diversity of this society in a vertical rather than a horizontal alignment, hardly surprising given that it is a diversity which he obviously regrets. This is particularly alarming, coming as it does from a man who is in charge of policing in one of the most metropolitan cities on earth. Newman, however, is blinded by a unitary model of "community" standards, derived from the unit of the family. That community values should vary can only be admitted to this scheme of things as evidence of *individual* faults and a loss of some essential moral unity which, it is felt, should encompass everybody across all divisions of class, race, gender and sexual orientation. What he is actually saying is very simple, though rather densely coded: the only good citizen is white, heterosexual, and in a family. And it is, of course, against marriage and the family that pornography is most frequently identified by most new right commentators. In this respect anti-pornography feminists such as Dworkin and MacKinnon, who favour local ordinances which ban pornography as a violation of women's rights, rather than an increase and extension of obscenity laws, are recruited notwithstanding to the cause of a politicised legal moralism which cannot but support patriarchal anti-gay values and institutions. In fact, as far as anti-pornography feminists are concerned, the notion that "violent images in films produce 'copycat' crimes in life has been documented"[25] is axiomatic, together with the desperate belief that women can only participate in pornography if they have either been forced or tricked in some way. This takes most models and actresses for fools, and is typical of a feminism which is endlessly searching for new ways to disavow the actual complexity and diversity of female sexuality, and to line up all women in an emotional bond of "sisterhood", which, as Angela Carter has argued, "is created by ignoring the disparate circumstances of social reality".[26] Thus feminism is co-opted to buttress the substantive sources of patriarchal power at the very moment in which it most eloquently mis-identifies that source as pornography. Writing in *New Socialist*, Susanne Kappeler takes up the fashionable cry:

> "Nobody knows where to draw the line, where pornography stops – because it doesn't stop anywhere. There is a smooth transition from the hard-core to the soft-core, to the photographic magazine to the advertisements, to literature and the arts".[27.]

But by this time any coherent notion of pornography, measured by content or effect, has been stretched out to the point of sheer meaninglessness. Even the generally prudent Rosalind Coward gives way on the subject to absurd biologistic generalisations about men and male power, attributing a "discharge view of sex" to all men, whereby, it would seem, "the male view of masturbation derives from a highly functional view of sex, a view which sees too much 'frustrated' desire as a bad thing, and 'release' from sexual tension as a good thing".[28] Similarly, sweeping statements about what "women" allegedly "like" and "don't like" hardly help matters, and are especially telling in the work of a writer who is generally, and elsewhere in this same article, admirably sensitive to questions of desire and fantasy, which refuse just the kind of over-simplified notions of what men or women "feel" about sex, which are so fervently peddled here. Such confusion suggests, of course, that we bring our own psychic as well as social histories to these debates, which tend to function in themselves like ritual purgings, with the enthusiasm of familiar anti-pornography "witness" muted only by considerations of liberal intellectual polemics. At the end of the day Coward wants us all to grow up and be "good" girls and "good" boys and stop playing with nasty, dirty toys. Like Kappeler, she extends the notion of pornography to include newspaper pin-ups, advertisements, anything in fact which may ever give any woman "offence". Together with a maddeningly prim and self-righteous tone, they both share the characteristic liberal feminist tendency to fudge over straightforward and crucial political issues of censorship and legal moralism, and further confuse the simple yet central distinction between coercive and consensual forms of sex, sliding endlessly between "representation" and "the real".

Hence the salutary and bracing effect of Beverley Brown's recommendation that we "lower the level of pornographic analysis"[29] rather than rush in to expand and elevate it. As she explains, pornography is a

"definite and limited cultural form with a specific mode of effectivity . . .merely characterising the pornographic in terms of explicitness is about as useful and as accurate as characterising capitalism as extreme misery".[30]

Her preferred analysis is aimed "in terms of pornography's mode of combining the components of genre, sexual fantasy and cultural objects." Brown begins her argument by noticing the agreement by liberals and non-liberals that "pornography can be characterised in terms of extremes of explicitness, that it is a matter of exposing to view certain acts or anatomies". Thus, pornography is presumed to contain a fixed content, along a spectrum of "extremes", involving both sexual behaviour and degrees of physical exposure, a presumption which implies the existence of a homogenous field of sexuality independent of, and available to, the workings of representation. Against this she protests "the distinctions of different forms of sexuality, in relation to which a concept of 'extreme' is simply unintelligible". Thus some sexual scenarios are deemed pornographic as the direct result of dress rather than undress, for example leather or bondage. What makes pornography distinguishable from medical photography

> "are its non-transparent features, the elements which constitute it as a distinctive representational genre – a certain rhetoric of the body, forms of narration, placing and wording of captions and titles, stylisations and postures, a repertoire of milieux and costume, lighting effects, etc."

The question is not whether or not pornography is "the" exemplary moment of patriarchy, but what sense we can make of sexual fantasy. Briskly dismissing feminist criticisms that pornography "objectifies" and "fragments" women's bodies, she points out "initially and tritely, all representation objectifies, all representation fragments". As she sees it, "the classic dilemma around pornography" involves "a balancing of extreme harms of doubtful direct connection with pornography against the harms censorship offers not only to traditionally conceived freedoms of the individual but now to feminist interests as well". In this context she also maintains the vital importance of not confusing different senses of "privacy", which is to be defended, for example in the sense of "not the law's business" with "in a private place" or "not exposed to view".

Beverley Brown clearly seeks to challenge a content-based theory of pornography with a generic approach, arguing that

> "the objects which pornography produces as erotic, in a form provocative to fantasy's tendency to accrete and solidify, are familiar objects. Insofar as fantasy does not work without material, there must be *some* object, arbitrary but not random. If that object is already connected with the sexual, so much the better. Pornography essentially provides a stock of visual repertoires constructed out of elements of the everyday, using objects, including elements of the feminine, already placed within definite cultural practices. In re-placing these objects, in making them available or special, as objects around which sexual fantasy can operate without too much wit or effort, pornography simultaneously opens up the possibility of a reversal, of seeing objects return to their cultural niches with a certain afterglow. Since pornography is concerned in constructing a form of recognisability or visibility for women within a space of eroticisation of everyday objects, it can have effects at the level of ordinary life without it having to make a long excursion by way of the 'extreme'; a day return will do, and do better."[31]

In this manner we can begin to think about the aggregation of sexual fantasy around objects of desire which are both socially local, and psychically general. Thus forbidden or censored desires can be smuggled into scenarios which are legitimated elsewhere within a culture according to non-sexual criteria, or at least according to criteria which do not recognise their own sexual investments – for example, the Wild West scenario so beloved of 1950s gay pornography, which will seem quite unobjectionable to non-gay spectators because they are finding other aspects of their identities in such imagery. Gay culture invariably works in this way on the pre-given *forms* of a heterosexual culture with its objects "re-placed", as Brown would put it, and homosexualised. The imagery of cowboys and Indians, inscribed throughout American national culture, is always ready and waiting, as it were, to "take up" other meanings, which read the relation between the two groups in quite a different light. Thus the movement of desire involving difference *within* the same sex is able to find ready-made instances of analogy within mainstream culture, and to make identifications with them, putting scenarios from heterosexual culture to new, unauthorised usage. At the same time it is important to remember that sexual identification on the part of gay men is always mobile, able to assume different roles and positions, which are always also power relations. "Content" and "effects" based approaches to pornography can never begin to consider the deeper question of how different pornographic images stand for different desiring subjects, or the terms on which fantasy identifications may be controlled or mobilised. This seems to me to be a *fundamental* aspect of pornography which is partially recognised but displaced into the rhetoric of harms by anti-pornography campaigners who are actually threatened by the possibility that they might "find themselves" within the eroticised space of a sexual fantasy scenario. The physical and verbal violence of anti-pornography campaigners of all persuasions certainly suggests that an unconscious defensive mechanism is vigorously at work to prevent any disturbance of consciousness. The violence of the response, its sheer excess, is then projected back onto the pornographic image itself. Harm has been done, but it is harm which took place in the unconscious during infancy and childhood, now rising dangerously near the surface of consciousness, not harm to a sexually formed individual.

In this respect most available theories of pornography amount to a kind of "false-consciousness" line or argument: sexual fantasies are held to be based on the direct "internalisation" of "misrepresentations". If these misrepresentations can only be set aside, and preferably locked away forever, then the entire system of sexuality might be magically transformed into the likeness of some techni-colour feminist Shangri-La, all tender, feeling, oceanic, tranquil – and deathlike. Thus the inevitable asymmetries of desire are tidily brushed away, out of sight and out of mind. Visual purity in this respect reflects a wider feminist culture in which physical "purity" is exalted, to the extent of calls for celibacy, or preferably "women-identified" relationships, which proceed not from sexual desire, but from shared psychological needs. It also speaks for the ancient discourse of cleansing the soul, cleansing the mind of "bad" thoughts. Power and desire are the two terms with which discussions of pornography should be framed, in an analysis of the actual *mise en scène* of individual images or narratives. To this task, notions of morality are simply distractive and irrelevant.

So, far from being a unitary phenomenon, recognisable from its explicit subject matter, pornography actually involves an immense array of what we might think of as "specialist literatures", each of which satisfies the sexual fantasy-structure of countless individuals, who thus find themselves addressed as a group in relation to the fantasy they share. Different "literatures" address and satisfy different groups. This is a level of sexual organisation which is entirely overlooked in a theory of sexuality which is mechanically rooted in distinctions between biological sex difference, and sexual object-choice. It is a level which organises individuals over and across all other divisions of class, gender, race, age and also sexual orientation. It is for this reason that a scenario of sexual fantasy – let's say a master/slave image – will be as ludicrous or pathetic to one pair of eyes as it is instinct with charged eroticism for another. Sexuality does not fix us into two immutable camps, consisting of male fantasisers and women as the objects of men's fantasies. Rather, we all move constantly between accepted and rejected identifications with one another, all the time, guided by desire. It is not pornography which is everywhere, it is fantasy.

What anti-pornography campaigners identify as "pornography" in a hierarchy of extremes is, in fact, merely the most direct and fixed expression of psychic processes which are omnipresent, either in the sexually projective way in which we all scan the world, or sublimated into the entire fabric of our everyday lives, lending pleasure to doing the ironing for one person, motivating the career as a photographer for another. As I have written elsewhere,

> "the discourse of pornography offers us 'good' sex and 'bad' sex, 'good' images and 'bad' images, 'good' dreams and 'bad' dreams. It collapses any possibility of considering how we actively negotiate all signs in our culture to make sense of

the world, into a crude picture of supposedly fixed universal meanings . . . The same discourse also makes it impossible to think about the ways in which we project our desires consciously and unconsciously all the time . . . awake or asleep. Desire informs every moment of our lives. Sexual desires do not simply lie inside words and images locked up like sardines in cans – rather they are determined by context, and by ceaseless mechanisms of displacement over which we have no conscious control. There is undoubtedly a task in making us aware of these processes, but it is not helped by imagining that we can ever finally arbitrate between signs which are 'sexual' and those which are not. To think otherwise is merely to take false consolation in self-deception".[32]

The notion of pornography thus reflects back only what anti-pornography campaigners already "know", either that sex is a unified system in which all men oppress all women by objectifying them, or that sex is a symbolic expression of the holy sacrament of marriage, not an occasion for lewd display and the celebration of carnality. As such it is *necessary* to the thought-structures of both mainstream feminism *and* religious or secular fundamentalism. In both instances the notion of pornography also proffers the delusion that sex is easily identified and contained. One sign of the re-homosexualisation of gay culture which I discussed in Chapter One may be found in the response of one gay man to a regular column in the *New York Native*, which prints supposedly "true-life" anecdotes about (mostly) casual sex:

> "It is editorially inconsistent and morally irresponsible to follow fifty pages of Aids reportage with the kind of pornography that Boyd McDonald serves up . . . Let's have a creative pornography constructed along lines other than power and the exchange of body fluids".[33]

This is the authentic voice of the feminist-identified gay man, spouting forth "on behalf" of other people perceived to be at risk, in terms which nonetheless perversely equate the possibility of HIV infection with quantitative rather than qualitative aspects of sex. This position might usefully be contrasted to a description of the video *Chance Of A Lifetime*, made by New York's Gay Man's Health Crisis, and encouraging Safer Sex, as "a pornographic healing". The fantasy scenarios in the video are immediately identifiable, and are directly targeted at groups defined by their mutual fantasy-structures, who are invited to "re-place" condoms into their particular field of sexual associations. This same video is, of course, totally illegal in the UK. Yet such materials remain the only means by which recalcitrant desire can be worked upon, at the level of fantasy itself, in order to encourage changes in sexual behaviour which are our only defence against the virus. Such laws were not called into being in order to prevent the dissemination of such materials. The fact remains, however, that the notion of a "pornographic healing" is profoundly inimical to the laws about representation in Britain, and would constitute no defence in court. As one American gay man wrote last year: "To hate porn is to hate sex. To hate sex is to hate being human. Porn tells us that sexuality is great, and, in the age of AIDS, that's a particularly important message to hear."[34]

Whilst it would hardly be consistent for me to call for a quasi legal banning of the use of the term "pornography", I nonetheless suggest that at the very least we should exercise the greatest caution in using it, and only then in order to challenge the validity of the entire debate which wells up behind it, whichever "side" one finds oneself on. We have clearer words with which to undertake the difficult task of analysing the workings of power in language and images. In this way we shall not be further contaminated by a discourse which can only identify us as perverts and agents of Satan or the patriarchy. I would thus suggest that it is ultimately pointless to assume an aggressive "pro-porn" stance, since the terms of any possible discussion have already been fixed in advance in such a way that we can only be heard as the voice of pornography itself, speaking in favour of actual sexual violence. The "pro-porn" position condemns one in any case to the hopeless roundabout of conflicting civil rights demands made on behalf of social constituencies which, by their very nature, can never be reconciled, either by rational means or legal *fiat*. What does matter is to continue to adopt a "pro- (safe) sex" position, to affirm the multiple erotic possibilities of our own bodies and other people's, and to challenge bigotry on our terms, rather than those supplied by the bigots.

Chapter Five

Aids and the press

In August, 1986, the *Los Angeles Times Magazine* published a "fictional scenario" entitled AIDS: 1991, "based on what is known about acquired immune deficiency syndrome".[1] The cover illustration shows a group of three featureless figures, with the suggestion of numbered identification tags around their necks, standing in a sombre limbo of swirling clouds of brown chalk. It is September, 1991, and "the White House has just announced that the Vice President's daughter and her five-month old son have Aids..." The number of Aids cases has reached 270,000, and one in every seventy American citizens have been infected by the HIV virus:

> "There are so many Aids patients that acute-care services at many hospitals have been in chronically short supply for years now. Insurance companies have been bankrupted. Every American is paying higher medical bills and insurance premiums... Nothing suggests that the general public, after years of denying that this 'gay plague' could affect them, knows enough to take the protective measures that would help to contain it."

A Presidential Commission calls for,

> "mandatory Aids testing of every US resident. Everybody will have to carry a photo identification card describing his or her test results. Those who are infected will be barred by law from having sex with uninfected people. Anyone found to have spread the infection will be jailed. Sex outside of marriage will be outlawed. Sodomy laws will be reinstated. If an infected woman becomes pregnant, she will be forced to have an abortion. Everyone entering the country – businessmen, tourists and Americans living abroad – will be quarantined for two weeks and then tested for the virus. All Americans will be tested for intravenous drugs, and drugusers will be forced into treatment programs or jailed... The whole world is beginning to consider the United States a diseased country."

Endorsing the Commission's recommendations, which seals all American borders in *both* directions, the president of the day informs the nation:

> "We have a crisis that requires drastic measures. Failure to follow these recommendations will undoubtedly lead to a need for even more drastic measures in the future ..."

The entire scenario of the article is set against two actual events in June, 1986 – the US Health Service's prediction of 250,000 cases of Aids within the next five years, and a legal opinion from the Justice Department that any employer could fire employees with Aids on suspicion that the virus could be spread in the workplace, regardless of medical evidence. (A majority of states have rejected this opinion, however, and adopted policies prohibiting discrimination against people with Aids.) Here, though, as is so frequently the case, Aids commentary is firmly fixed in the future tense, in this instance borrowing a speculative apocalyptic form from science fiction. This is presumably intended to force back pressure onto the present, in the form of preventative state action. What is so alarming, however, across the entire spectrum of printed commentary, is the inability to conceive of Aids in the *present*, as it is experienced world-wide by millions of people. All the policies envisaged take for granted the effectiveness and desirability of interventions by criminal law in relation to both disease and sexuality, as if Aids – and, by extension, homosexuality – could be legislated off the face of the earth. What is more, these measures are accepted uncritically as both workable and necessary in the face of the sheer enormity of the fictive catastrophe described. A future is thus framed in such a way that possibilities are pushed nearer probability, with a familiar obsession over quantitative rather than qualitative aspects of sexual behaviour. Quarantine emerges as a "thinkable" strategy from the direct force of the narrative, and its resemblance to stories we already know from television, cinema and popular fiction – stories of holocaust, disaster and annihilation. The Californian reader is thus "lined up" in relation to the then forthcoming LaRouche Initiative, which upheld a strict quarantine policy towards people with Aids, and was due to go to the ballot box three months after the article was published.

Throughout the article we read an implication of collective guilt on the part of those indulging in sexual activity outside marriage, a guilt which focuses most sharply on those who in any case are not legally entitled to marry one another, namely gay men, whose morality is judged against familial standards and, of course, is found wanting. In this way a particularly impractical and unjust policy proposal is floated before its potential electorate as a voice of sanity speaking on behalf of national security and even national survival. That the quarantining of everyone testing positive in California would cost 7.9 billion dollars, one quarter of the state's annual budget,[2] is hardly to be considered when the agenda is exclusively moralistic. Nor do financial considerations matter when the policy involved is less important than establishing a general sense of imminent social peril for wider political purposes. In any case, referendum politics have to be extremely carefully orchestrated, since they tend to take their potential supporters for more or less gullible fools. The more didactic the tone, the lower the turn-out at the polls. Thus a recent referendum in Augusta, Maine, which would have made it illegal to sell or possess "sex toys and materials containing explicit sex descriptions or photographs" was defeated by a margin of more than two to one.[3]

In contemporary America, "land of the profit-making casualty ward, home of the taxi-metered ambulance",[4] most Aids commentary in the press turns a stubborn, Nelson-like blind eye to the situation of all people with Aids whose illness cannot be readily recruited to the cause of "protecting" the "innocent". That thousands of people with Aids have already been pauperised by the illness, that they will "encounter the suspicion and contempt that America traditionally accords to its poor",[5] that in New York City (where the epidemic is now the leading cause of death for white males aged between twenty and forty) there is no out-patient care and hospitals are turning people away daily, is simply beyond the range of vision of the mainstream commercial newspaper and periodical industry. Acute care services in many American hospitals are already in chronically short supply. Insurance companies have refused to offer policies to gay men who have not taken the HIV test with negative results. Nothing suggests that Safer Sex information is getting through to people outside the urban gay communities and their immediate constituents. Sodomy laws have been reinstated. The worst does not need to be projected onto the year 1991: for many millions of people it has already happened, and is an inescapable fact of life. Hence the need to understand how "the worst" is conceived, and on whose terms.

The key word here, in relation both to homosexual desire and a disease now innately identified with it, is *projection*, which Leo Bersani describes as "a frantic defence against the return of dangerous images and associations to the surfaces of consciousness", a process whereby it is urgently maintained "that certain representations or affects belong to the world and not to the self".[6] It is from this perspective that I will consider the work of Aids commentary in the press, since the organisation and evaluation of this commentary does not obey the apparent distinction between tabloid and quality publications, any more than it operates within the alignments of party politics. In this respect Aids reportage tells us far more about journalism than it does about Aids. Thus in Britain we find the leading style and fashion magazine *The Face* piously informing us that,

> "the Moral Majority view that it is a reward for two decades of increasing sexual license, a plague on gays, has disturbed deep-rooted fears. The AIDS scare has reinvested a fashionable, almost mundane homosexuality with taboo, rendered it marginal again. Despite the frank admissions and frantic gender-bending of pop stars in the not-so-gay Eighties, acceptance of homosexuality has now joined the other liberal causes in retreat... The spectre of the decade: Transmission Electron Micrograph of stages in the growth of Human T-Cell Leukemia Virus 111, identified as the cause of AIDS".[7]

This is printed only half legibly in white against a double-page enlargement, together with appropriately "scientific" looking charts of incidence, the words of the text dissolving into the image of the virus, which stares out like a huge eye. Whilst *The Face*'s public profile is invariably liberal to left of centre on questions of race and governmental politics, it has nonetheless sustained a low level but persistent tenor of homophobia since its inception, in its early years providing a regular platform for arch-homophobic journalist Julie Burchill to spout her particular brand of suburban-chic prejudice. The "deep-rooted" fears which Aids has supposedly "disturbed" are evidently in the mind of the writer, and if anything "frantic" is going on, it is his (or her) fantasy of a "fashionable, almost mundane homosexuality". What we are witnessing is an attempt to push homosexuality back from a public sphere which it has never inhabited, save in the eyes of the law and other institutional guardians of moral "welfare", including journalism.

Such commentary clearly disavows the social reality of Aids in the strict sense of disavowal, defined as,

> "a mode of defence which consists in the subject's refusing to recognise the reality of a traumatic perception... Inasmuch as disavowal affects *external reality*, Freud sees it as the first stage of psychosis, and he opposes it to repression: whereas the neurotic starts by repressing the demands of the id, the psychotic's first step is to disavow reality".[8]

We find a similar mechanism at work in the *Daily Mail*, where the reliably homophobic correspondent George Gordon describes an America

> "gripped with fear, loathing and hysteria over the relentless increase of the unexplained killer disease AIDS. What is terrifying its leaders is that the national mood is only a twitch away from focusing that hysteria onto a human target – the millions of gay men who until now have flaunted their 'gayness' before the straight society ... When Rock Hudson admitted he had AIDS, the gay community exploited the fact with near joy. At last they had a public figure, a hero who was one of them. The biggest name in AIDS. The reality has been that it has focused attention on AIDS and also on the causes of it. The gay parades are over. So too is public tolerance of a society that paraded its sexual deviance and demanded rights. The public is now demanding to live disease-free with the prime carriers in isolation".[9]

It should by now, I hope, be clear that it is Gordon who is "gripped with fear, loathing and hysteria". The term hysteria covers a wide class of neuroses, of which, according once more to Laplanche and Pontalis,

> "the two best isolated forms, from the point of view of symptoms, are *conversion hysteria*, in which the psychical conflict is expressed symbolically in somatic symptoms of the most varied kinds: they may be paroxystic (e.g., emotional crises accompanied by theatricality) or more long-lasting (anaesthesias, hysterical paralyses, 'lumps in the throat', etc.); and *anxiety hysteria*, where the anxiety is attached in more or less stable fashion to a specific external object (phobias)".[10]

Hence the astonishingly casual way in which Gordon reattributes his own sickening exploitation of the death of Rock Hudson back onto a supposedly unified "gay community", all the more terrifying to him since he recognises that he is not just talking about a few "weirdos", but about millions of adult Americans, a constituency immensely larger than the readership of the *Daily Mail*. In one sentence Aids is "unexplained", but by the end of his piece he knows "the causes of it", at which point he moves into hysterical super-drive, completely unable to distinguish his own wishes from reality, for the gay parades are far from over. The problem is evidently not that lesbians and gay men "demanded rights", but that throughout the United States they campaigned and fought for and *won* them. In a final flourish of phobic delusion he dresses up as "the public" itself, in a hygienic fantasy of mass-quarantine (where? how?) with barely concealed genocidal overtones. For the only explanation of regarding all gay men as killers, the "cause" and source of Aids, is a displaced desire to kill them all – the teeming deviant millions – oneself. Or, better still, to get the readers of the *Daily Mail* to do it for you. Gordon's letters from America regularly smoulder with this degree of pathological anxiety concerning homosexuality, which he seems to regard as an American phenomenon, from which Britain can and must somehow be protected.

Incitement to violence against gay men is a regular aspect of British press coverage of our lives. Thus, after a particularly unpleasant sexual assault on a small boy in Brighton, the *Sun*'s front page headline screamed "GAYS IN FEAR: They dread revenge after attack on boy". The *Sun* is hardly siding with vulnerable gay men here: it is calling out for anti-gay violence, in a direct if crude discourse of revenge.[11] Hence the significance of the two framing stories which report "Three Hurt In Pub Shooting" and "I Saw Guard Shot Dead By Bandits". By means of such chains of association on a single page, meanings are anchored and intentions signified, consciously or otherwise. The reporting of Aids is thus inexorably caught up in the larger discourse of retribution against gay men, which both precedes and exceeds the unfolding of the epidemic. That this has contributed to such widespread ignorance and misconception about Aids, and put newspaper readers at real risk, is one of the more glaring ironies of Aids journalism.

Most newspapers depend on advertising revenue for their economic survival. It is thus their business to address an audience of readers as potential consumers for the commodities which they advertise. Moving between the spheres of domesticity, work and leisure, the press is no longer tied directly to political parties, and makes its primary appeal to "the family", seen both as the central site of *economic* consumption, in the form of clothes, cosmetics, furniture, holidays and so on, as well as a primarily *moral* entity, since it also occupies the space of sexuality and child-raising. Many newspapers are in any case themselves part of larger corporate conglomerates which produce the very products which they test, review and advertise. "The family" is thus positioned in newspaper discourse as the central term of professional journalistic know-how, establishing a fixed agenda of values, interests and concerns which are heavily moralised, to the virtual exclusion of all other approaches. Moreover, given that most people do not in fact live in households which conform to received images of family life, this involves a considerable degree of fantasy on the part of journalists and readers alike. Nonetheless, newspapers claim to represent "the family" against anyone who threatens its sovereignty, from governments to "busy-body social workers".

Thus in the *Daily Mail* we read that,

> "Family is a sexist word – because it discriminates against homosexuals and lesbians. That is the verdict of a working party set up by Labour-ruled Lambeth Council in South London... The working party – which includes homosexual and trade union co-opted members – says the word family is 'generally assumed to mean heterosexual adults with children'. The suggested alternative is 'households with children'... Talks are to go ahead with local magistrates to encourage the adoption of children by homosexual and lesbian couples. And the council is expected to accept the... recommendation to encourage the recruitment of homosexual child-minders... Homosexual couples look like being offered homes on the same basis as heterosexuals."

All this is neatly rounded off with a quote from the then GLC leader, Ken Livingstone, reportedly saying that "some people are actively homosexual, others aren't. It depends on what happens to you in your early life".[12] In a sense this is true, but in this context Livingstone's description of sexual diversity is simply recruited to the notion of homosexuality as a threat to children, and itself the product of sexual interference in childhood. Here, as in countless thousands of similar articles, the reader is invited to rally to the rescue of the poor little defenceless word "family", as well as its poor little defenceless child members, in the face of a homosexuality which is not merely lurking in the garden, but waiting to come indoors with council authority. Thus the press prioritises the stigmatisation of homosexuality above all other issues, since it is here that the national family unit is held to be most united, though paradoxically also most in need of regular reminders of the risks they are perpetually running. In the name of defending "privacy", any amount of legislation which directly affects and regulates the internal life of the household is called for and actively supported. At the same time, a framework of "popular memory" is accumulated, in which the patriarchal white heterosexual nation is forever seen as the victim of dramatic crimes and assaults which stimulate the most basic levels of homophobic anxiety. Newspapers traumatise their readers steadily and with care: the *People* advertises itself on television as the paper "that will shake you". But far from shaking inward-looking, narrow familial identities open in order to acknowledge diversity, newspapers, in fact, confine them ever more rigorously within the rigid and obsessive narratives of sexual scandal and xenophobic patriotism. The "general public" thus emerges as a highly abstract category, which is united across all divisions of class, age, party political affiliations, and gender, by recourse to extremely narrow moral criteria. Thus the press will always defend "privacy", which it pictures as constantly beleaguered, whilst at the same time it calls for ever increasing regulation of the home. Only parental adult sexuality is encouraged, whilst sexuality outside the family emerges as its most serious adversary.

Newspapers also offer themselves as national publications, though, in fact, they are invariably regional in origin and focus. The press champions national identity as a sense of personal value, establishing a whole series of analogies between the security of the family and that of the nation. The sense of loyalty to one's newspaper thus feeds off other loyalties, which in turn are identified with it. This national identity is also, like "the family", presented as highly vulnerable, and is similarly established in terms of supposedly fixed and innate characteristics, resulting from "breeding". In this manner the newspaper constructs an ideal audience of national family units, surrounded by the threatening spectacle of the mad, the foreign, the criminal and the perverted. The press is therefore heavily dependant upon the very categories which it ceaselessly offers up as exemplary signs of "the breakdown of law and order" or simply "the disgusting" or "the depraved". Scandal serves the purpose of exemplary exclusion in newspaper discourse, and is the central means whereby readers find themselves reassured and reconciled as "normal", law-abiding citizens. Hence the remorseless diet of racism and homophobia.

In a professional sense, "good" journalism therefore consists in persuading the newspaper reading audience to recognise itself with pleasure and reassurance as individual members of a white patriarchal "general public", whose values and institutions must at all costs be regarded as threatened rather than threatening. Hence the spectacle endlessly repeated at film premieres and Royal Weddings and Presidential primaries, of the powerful and privileged congratulating one another in the public space of the newspaper, before the grovellingly grateful and adoring eyes of those who know and accept their own social inferiority. This is the world where "men are men" and "women are women", and the British press is proudly and erroneously proclaimed as the "freest" in the world. These fixed categories of gender, race, class, sexuality and national identity, and all their myriad derivations, are orchestrated together in order to protect readers from the actual diversity of social and sexual life, which it is also the business of the press stridently to denounce as immoral, indecent and unnatural.

Thus "the scandalous" is firmly structured as that which transgresses against the coherence of one or more of these categories, that which flouts their validity and must therefore be exposed. Homosexuality is a permanent scandal, like child sexuality and republicanism. The merest possibility of a contingency linking Royalty to homosexuality guarantees a "good story", as demonstrated by the *Star* with a recent front page banner headline: "GAY LOVERS ON ROYAL YACHT: Shock as Fergie and Andrew plan honeymoon". This appeared as a "*Star* Exclusive" not long before the wedding in London of Prince Andrew and Sarah Ferguson. We read that,

> "Gay sailors have been serving the Queen and Prince Philip aboard the Royal Yacht *Britannia*, the *Star* can exclusively reveal. The scandal came to light when steward Keith Jury told his wife he'd been having an affair with a Royal Marine Bandsman"

and so on. This "story" is stretched out to a full three pages, with another banner headline draped across the top of pages two and three proclaiming: "Goodbye Sailor! I'm divorcing gay sailor says Gillian", above an unkind photograph of "The Wife He Left Behind". In an accompanying interview she states:

> "we had a wonderful marriage until he joined that ship ... I still can't seem to think that this happened. There was nothing abnormal about him or our sex life. After all, we have three children."

and then, in italics,

> *"he was a bit effeminate, I suppose, but I thought it was just his manner ... not anything like this."*[13]

Here we find the familiar "hybridised" picture of homosexuality, at once virile and masculine ("we have three children"), and now feminised and enfeebled ("I thought it was just his manner ..."). But most important of all is the sense of a far more scandalous possibility which emerges from the contingency of gay men and the newlyweds, namely Aids. This is nowhere directly articulated in the story, but is the inevitable conclusion readers will reach by the sheer overlap of narratives about homosexuality, Aids and the monarchy. Aids is the missing yet crucial term which "explains" the otherwise inexplicable length of the story in the first place. In this way the mere fact of gay sex is held to be dangerous for other people, not as a temptation to imitate, but as a hazard to life itself. And this slippage, from "gay" to

h" is by now a commonplace of Aids commentary in
re-connecting an alignment between homosexuality
hich Wolfenden Strategy had all but undone.

thus radically prescriptive. It presents the world
ke to see in the likeness of an imaginary national
past, just as it defends and justifies its rejection of what it cannot
acknowledge in the present by recourse to imaginary futures. And
when the contour maps of sexuality and national identity are obliged
to duplicate one another, it is homosexuality which is squeezed out
first. This mapping operation can only accept one primary distinction
between human subjects – the physical opposition male/female.
Other divisions which threaten to disrupt and invalidate this picture
are ruthlessly stigmatised. Thus the hospital ward joins the prison cell
as the "proper" site of homosexuality, offering a limited and closely
supervised window onto the forbidden and unknown, and finding
there what it consistently warned against all along – corruption and
contagion – the just deserts of those who are thought to reject the
national family. In a situation where sexuality and gender are clearly
held as the primary determinations of "character", in a discourse of
"real men" and "real women", gay men and lesbians are serious
offenders. Thus the press "knows" what its readers are like, in
relation to the pivotal roles of family life – "mums", "dads", "kids",
even "pets", which act out all the other roles "in little" as it were. All
these characters have regularly coded appearances, inflected by class,
and their combinations are equally predictable in advance, constituted in a continuum of expectations which stretches from
cartoons and gossip columns through regular sections on gardening,
sports, finance, fashion, and so on. Homosexuality can only enter this
space as an intrusion, just as gay culture in all its forms will be given
the spurious unity of a criminal environment, an infernal and bestial
domain which is virtually non-human.

What so distinguishes the treatment of Aids has been the constant
inability to offer any possibility of identification with the vast
majority of those most closely affected by the illness. Viewed as
illegitimate national subjects, the state of our health is of no more
interest than our lives, unless they can provide yet more evidence of
our fundamentally *alien* status. A disease of cats or hamsters would
have attracted more sympathy for its sufferers, and their contingent
human owners, than has Aids. I am not aware of a single article in the
mainstream British press which pays serious attention to the situation
of the two million or so gay men in the UK who are currently living
through this crisis with varying degrees of courage, grief, fear and
stress. All that is most sordid and guilt-ridden in "official" British
culture is projected away onto the relatively benign and balanced

sexual egalitarianism of lesbians and gay men, in an astonishing torrent of anxiety concerning bodies and sex. Construing us as ruthless perverts, failed heterosexuals, half-men and half-women, homophobic reporting is able to draw deeply from the brackish wells of nationalistic chauvinism, combining a lively anti-intellectualism with a profound terror of sex in all its forms, which is the particularly unhappy legacy of puritanism.

All this is lined up on huge public hoardings concerning "standards", "decency" and, above all, "respectability", which claim absolute, universal and incontrovertible validity. Thus the *Sun* announces the introduction of two gay men to the most popular national television soap opera, *EastEnders*, with the front page headline: "It's Eastbenders: Gay Men Stir Up TV Soap". Their reporter tells us,

> "*EastEnders* is turning into Eastbenders... with two gays joining the TV soap's line-up. Designer Colin Russell, played by hunky actor Michael Cashman, will move into Tony Carpenter's Albert Square flat to live with a male lover – And one *EastEnders'* insider said last night 'Like it or not, gays are part of the community... Obviously an over-the-top drag artist doesn't reflect what the average gay man is like... We hope to show viewers that homosexual males are not necessarily limp-wristed and effeminate'... There is no suggestion that actor Michael Cashman is gay in real life. He is simply playing a role."[14]

There is evidently no sense of contradiction between the headline's evaluation of the "story", the "insider's" information, and the closing remark. Yet again, the fact of sexual diversity is folded back into a larger and more powerful discourse of phobic embarrassment, leaving the pejorative word "bender" to suppress other rival meanings which have been put into play. This is reinforced by the pathological insistence that the actor is distinct from the part he plays, as if to reassure readers that no actor who is gay in "real life" could possibly appear on *EastEnders*, the focal point of early evening family entertainment.

It is from this perspective that we should regard the coverage of Rock Hudson's death, which offered journalists an opportunity for particularly vicious revenge on a man whom they had casually taken to embody their own patriarchal and misogynistic values for more than three decades. To begin with we should note the practical impossibility of Hudson's "coming out" as gay in the American film industry of the 1950s, when he was at the height of his fame, given the intensely homophobic atmosphere of McCarthyite values in Hollywood. At the same time, Hudson's starring roles in films such as *Written On The Wind*, *Magnificent Obsession*, and especially *All That Heaven Allows*, construct him as a figure quite removed from mainstream macho 1950s masculinity, as represented by Victor Mature or Clarke Gable. On the contrary, Hudson's film persona frequently presented him as a "sensitive" figure, a "gentle giant", aligned with nature rather than masculine culture.

On 24 July, 1985, the *Mirror*'s headline announced "Rock Hudson AIDS Fear: 'Very, very sick man'", with a before-and-after comparison invited between two photographs. The day after his death the *Daily Mail* headline recorded "The Last Days Of Rock Hudson: He died a living skeleton – and so ashamed", whilst the commentary stated that Hudson, "Hollywood's macho sex symbol who unknown to his millions of women fans was a secret homosexual, died yesterday of AIDS". On page three, another headline informs us "Hollywood made the legend, Rock Hudson lived the lie".[15] On the same day the *Sun* repeated the same approach, with a double page title in a huge typeface, "The Hunk Who Lived A Lie: He loved only Mum", describing Hudson as "the original Hollywood hunk" who,

> "played out the fantasies of millions of men as he kissed and caressed some of the world's most beautiful women. But the Romeo driven by passion on film could not love any of these sexy screen goddesses – because he was gay... Thankfully the only woman he ever loved – his mother, Kay – never lived to know her son had AIDS".

Just by comparing these two accounts, it emerges that the central focus of Hudson's death concerns firstly a denunciation of "dishonesty", secondly a "betrayal" of male and female fans' fantasies, and thirdly the imputation of a guilty sense of responsibility for their illness to people with Aids. Hence the relief with which the *Sun* notes that Hudson's mother "thankfully" "never lived to know her son had AIDS".[16] It is clearly impossible for the *Sun* to recognise that death is not automatically and necessarily preferable to acknowledging that a close relative is gay. It is equally – and still more culpably – impossible for the journalist to acknowledge that hundreds of parents are actually supporting gay sons and their lovers through Aids. The role of the press in "shaming" the parents of gay people with Aids is perhaps the single most nauseating aspect of Aids commentary.

The *Mirror* also took up the theme of "A Soul in Torment", headlining "The tragic double life of a macho movie star", and describing Hudson "doing his embroidery" at an interview:

> "There he was, all six-foot-five of him, complete with an inch-deep tan, a vast smile and shoulders the width of a lorry... 'Don't you think this is pretty?' he growled in his bassoon voice."[17]

Here Hudson has to be dramatically feminised in order to cancel out the sheer scale of the opening image. And the *Star* reported "Women adored him... but his macho image was a sordid sham: The Heart-Throb Who Lived A Lie",[18] following earlier reporting patterns, brought in from America: "Day One Of An Exclusive Star Series: Living A Lie".[19] As Michel Foucault, who also died as a result of Aids, observed in an interview, "to call homosexuals liars is equivalent to calling the resistors under military occupation liars. It's like calling Jews 'money-lenders' when it was the only profession they were allowed to practise".[20] It is a peculiarly obnoxious strategy in the mouth of an industry which scrupulously ensures the discursive pathologising and criminalisation of homosexual desire in all its forms and manifestations. Summing up the year's news at Christmas, the *Daily Mail* printed the familiar before-and-after shots of Hudson's face, with the pointed text, "The two faces of Hollywood – vibrant, virile... dissipated, corrupt, decadent – captured on the two faces of Rock Hudson, the first celebrity victim of AIDS".[21] But a single image is still more telling of press commentary and practices. It shows the interior of a transit van, with a man inside shielding his face, and something wrapped up on a stretcher. Beneath a caption "Body taken off in a van" we are told that this is "the body of Rock Hudson" in "a sealed bag"...

> "There was no Hollywood glitter as the body was taken away from Hudson's Beverley Hills mansion within hours of his death. Only a small crowd of fans watched as it was driven off to a secret location, where he was cremated. A friend of the star said: 'Rock had requested that he be cremated as soon as possible after his death.'"[22]

What we were not told, however, was that in fact

> "the order to cremate the star's remains so quickly came from his closest friends after they learned magazines were offering £50,000 for a picture of the self-confessed homo-sexual".[23]

A scrummage of photographers had torn open the back of the transit van, with all the due respect they habitually offer to easy money.

In the regulatory codes of Aids reportage Rock Hudson remains hot news, as a *Sun* Exclusive a year later bears out, with the headline

"Madonna Buys Rock's Plague Palace". Apparently "the original asking price was £6 million. But that was slashed to the half-price bargain offer because it was on the market for more than ten months during the big AIDS scare in America".[24] The last word in hypocrisy, however, should go to the *Daily Mail*, with its suggestion that "the tension caused by his years of living a lie may indeed have contributed to his heavy drinking and his heart trouble, culminating in emergency by-pass surgery in 1981".[25] Not content with blaming Hudson for his own death, the *Mail* puts into effect a final reversal whereby he was also morally responsible for other illnesses in his life, which are understood to stem from a personal "problem" of his own making, rather than the concerted vicious homophobia of the press industry. All this is a far and sorry cry away from the dominant tenor of American press coverage, which even in the depths of Baptist Oklahoma could record "Hudson Saluted For His Courage", printing an Associated Press story which begins with a very different picture of the actor as "a 'white knight in shining armour' whose courage in acknowledging before he died that he had AIDS may be the catalyst that spurs worldwide efforts to find a cure".[26]

Writing rather strangely in the past tense, Frances FitzGerald has described in the *New Yorker* how

> "of all the modern epidemic diseases, AIDS was in many respects the most terrible. In the first place, the mean incubation period for AIDS (as was later discovered) was about five years. This meant that a victim could have the virus anywhere from a few months to as long as fourteen years before the first symptoms (such as fatigue, glandular swellings, and weight loss) manifested themselves, and during that time it was altogether possible that he or she could infect others without knowing it. Once AIDS was diagnosed, the victim might have six months, a year, even three or four years to live, but virtually no-one had survived for more than five years. Since there was no cure, the victim simply had to await the onset of one or more diseases that his system could not fight off... As AIDS moved relatively slowly through the body, so it moved relatively slowly through the population. And in this respect it was also excruciating."[27]

This I take as fairly typical American reporting of the epidemic. It certainly acknowledges the nightmarish reality in which thousands of people find themselves in America, yet it still manages to contain them as "victims", totally passive, and unable to do anything but sit around waiting to die. Thus, as Edmund White concludes with reference to the American press,

> "our communitarian tradition has caused us to think of gays
> as an ethnic group like any other. This conception is surely
> the main reason for the earlier strength of Gay Liberation
> and the current efficacy of gay pressure groups. But a ghetto
> is not only a community center; it's also a good target for a
> pogrom. If gays are 'a race apart', then they can be subjected
> to racism".[28]

Nonetheless, Frances FitzGerald's comments should alert us to the
plain stupidity and complex sadism involved in attempts to "blame"
individuals for "passing on" a virus which they didn't even know to
exist. And even now, when much more is known about the disease,
information about Safer Sex is hardly easy to come by, even for urban
gay men who regularly visit bars and discos.

It is in this context that we should attend to what are presented as
more "scholarly" types of commentary, as served up, for example, in
neo-conservative periodicals such as *The American Spectator* where,
after initial rhetorical flourishes indicting government inaction, we
are told that "we should be studying the epidemiology of AIDS
scientifically, not sociologically, for without proper information we
will not have rational action".[29] Lurking not far behind this tired
fantasy of scientific disinterestedness, and much blinding with
spurious scientific analogies, we get to the heart of the matter, or
rather the rectum, since Aids here is directly attributed to
"promiscuous sodomy". Campaigns for Safer Sex information are
arrogantly brushed aside in a manner which is only surprising until
one realises that they threaten the central drift of the article, which
concludes that "from what we know now the only alternative
available until cures or vaccines ... are developed, is to prevent the
spread of the disease by making it physically impossible. This implies
strict quarantine..." Given the very epidemiological nature of Aids,
however, it is clear that quarantining people with opportunistic
infections would hardly make a halfpenny-worth of difference, and
one can only read such appeals as either displaced vengeance or, more
cynically, as straightforward homophobic recruitment material for
the new right, substituting "gay men" for "niggers" in a politics of
fear.

Either explanation, or both, might apply to reports like that in the
Times which explained that

> "at present, a network of promiscuous urban homosexual-
> ity, constantly folding back on itself, provides an ideal
> diffusion field for any infection getting into it. Recent tests

on a group of promiscuous but quite fit New York
homosexuals revealed that eighty per cent were suffering
some kind of immune disturbance".[30]

Was there a comparative test of "promiscuous" heterosexuals?
Answer comes there none. Hence the widespread tendency to
distinguish between "innocent" and "guilty" victims, the former
consisting of babies, married women and so on, the latter gay men
who, it is constantly implied, should have somehow "known better",
the phrase used by *Observer* journalist Annabel Ferriman at the first
British conference on the subject of Aids and the media.[31] The science
correspondent for the same paper, Robin McKie, is still able to write
of a recent survey in Manhattan that "the study shows Aids is
spreading with alarming speed through American cities where it is
establishing itself as a heterosexual disease".[32] That diseases do not
have desires seems not to have occurred to him, and it is the repetition
of just this type of unconscious assumption which defines the profile
of Aids reporting at its most pernicious and inadequate.

The worst examples of Aids coverage I have come across are not
the explicitly homophobic which are relatively transparent, though
sickening, but the more subtle "human interest" stories. Thus the
cover of *Woman's Own* proclaims: "This baby's got AIDS! Read his
mother's tragic story". Inside, one Simon Kinnersley introduces us to
the Zozup family from the suburbs of Washington, USA – baby
Mathew, and parents Sue and Steve, neither of whom "had ever taken
any drugs" and "didn't drink much for that matter either, nor had
they had many affairs let alone relationships with homosexuals".[33]
Note the "let alone". Mathew's life "is a harsh and vivid reminder
that Acquired Immune Deficiency Syndrome is no longer only the
'gay plague'". Note again the "only", and the implication that, after
all, a "gay plague" is what we're really talking about. Mathew was a
premature baby, and as he "lay in his incubator undergoing the tests
and blood transfusions necessary because of his early arrival,
someone reached out and touched that defenceless new-born child
with death". Here the image of "gay plague" is personalised into the
vampire-like image of intentional murder. In this manner a terrible
tragedy is recruited to the wider purposes and values of homophobia.
Commenting on the television film *An Early Frost*, the baby's mother
is reported to have said:

"I've got nothing against the homosexual community...
because knowing what AIDS is like I wouldn't wish it on any
human being, but they were consenting adults, they *did* have
a choice".

And "as she talks, her voice trembles and tears well up in her eyes". That *"did"* is the only italicised word in the entire article, and carries the crucial weight of distinguishing "innocent" from "guilty", pushing responsibility back clearly and unambiguously onto gay men in general and, as we have seen, onto one in particular.

A still more repulsive piece from the same Simon Kinnersley appeared only two months later, once more in *Woman's Own*. This time the cover prepared us for "The sad, sad story of the woman with AIDS".[34] This story concerns Sunnye Sherman, from Silver Springs, Washington DC:

> "No-one ever told her that sleeping with a man could be like facing a firing squad ... no-one said that sex – normal, healthy, conventional sex – could kill. Nor did they warn her that it would be a slow and painful end, filled with suffering, almost constant agony and illness. That she would enter a twilight world from which death, when it came, would be a welcome relief".

Sunnye was infected unwittingly by her bisexual fiancé and, having lost her own job, worked as an Aids counsellor. Kinnersley writes that "she still feels no bitterness, no hatred and no loathing towards the man who actually gave her AIDS", which he evidently finds impossible to believe, allowing the repetition of "bitterness", "hatred" and "loathing" to do his dirty work for him. Nor, of course, did anyone "give Aids" to Sunnye, or to anyone else, since Aids itself cannot be transmitted. It is a syndrome, not an infection. This terribly simple yet vital point is entirely lost on Kinnersley, and the vast majority of his colleagues. Sunnye is still friends with the man concerned. As she points out,

> "it was so long ago, we knew nothing about AIDS, we showed all the correct responsibility for what we knew at the time. I knew he was bisexual, but as far as we were both concerned the only danger was getting pregnant, and I took care of that ... it was a joint responsibility and choice".

Since this clearly snatches the axe which Mr Kinnersley wants so much to grind from his hands, he is forced to look for other means. Thus we read that,

> "as she prepares to die, Sunnye casts a cold eye at the casual attitude that she, like so many other people, had towards sex".

Kinnersley evidently knew all along that sex is dangerous. When Sunnye is allowed to speak for herself, she states to the contrary that she,

> "would like to think that because of what's happened to
> people like me, others will be more careful. It might not
> sound very romantic discussing what sort of sexual diseases
> your proposed lover has had, or whether he's had a blood
> transfusion, taken drugs intravenously and, if he's bisexual,
> has he had the HTLV3 (AIDS blood) test, but you have to
> remember that your life could depend on it."

This is good sense, and betrays none of the rabid moralism or
homophobia which are so typical of the Kinnersley school of
journalism.

At this moment in time, everything to do with Aids is
newsworthy. That is to say, Aids is caught up in the larger machine of
sales wars and takeover battles within the newspaper industry. And in
sales terms Aids is "good" news. Hence we find stories being invented
from scratch which sustain public alarm at a high level of profitability
to the newspaper owners. Thus we find the *Sun* sending out its
reporter Peter Cliff to report on "My Misery Posing As AIDS Victim:
Why the country closed its doors on me".[35] Cliff travelled round
Britain telling people he was an "AIDS victim" as he asked for
haircuts, dental treatment, hotel rooms and so on. A taxi driver, Steve
Bowen, is shown in a photograph rejecting our redoubtable reporter,
saying: "I can't take you, mate. I can't afford the risk. My wife has
just had a daughter and if I took money from your hands I don't
know what I could pass on". An unfortunate Scottish housewife
whom Cliff accosted:

> "looked at me in horror when I asked the way to the nearest
> clinic and told her I was suffering from the disease. She took
> to her heels and screamed over her shoulder: 'Don't come
> near me'".

Perhaps she recognised him as a man from the *Sun*. Against all this
preposterous nonsense is a tiny list of examples of "The Few Who
Cared" and, tucked away at one side, "The Truths Behind The
Myths", which is clear and accurate, and has the telephone number of
The Terrence Higgins Trust. But if the *Sun* were seriously concerned
about how people with Aids are treated in contemporary Britain, why
didn't they ask some? The answer lies, I think, in the fact that the *Sun*
cannot finally permit the possibility of humanising the epidemic, or
allowing gay men to appear in any other terms than those prepared
for them by the phobic and fearful gentlemen of the press.

Still more bizarre was the *Sun*'s earlier story headlined "I'd Shoot
My Son If He Had AIDS, Says Vicar!: He would pull trigger on rest

of his family".[36] Described as "Another red hot *Sun* exclusive", this piece concerns the Reverend Robert Simpson, who "vowed yesterday that he would take his teenage son to a mountain and shoot him if the boy had the deadly disease AIDS". Both of them obligingly stepped outside to have their picture taken, which appears above a caption which reads "Shotgun message... The Rev Robert Simpson demonstrates his point about AIDS with the help of son Chris". It is an extraordinary image of a man holding a rifle at a boy at point-blank range. It is also the very image of everything the press fears most – family breakdown, infanticide, teenage sexuality, homosexuality – printed approvingly as a warning image. The Rev Simpson said

> "he would ban all practising homosexuals, who are most in danger of catching AIDS, from taking normal communion... If it continues it will be like the Black Plague. It could wipe out Britain. Family will be against family".

And he "calls on the Government to repeal the law on homosexuality between consenting adults and prostitution – and to punish promiscuity".

In the face of all this gibberish, it is immediately helpful to turn to Freud's concept of the return of the repressed, a process whereby

> "what has been repressed – though never abolished by repression – tends to reappear, and succeeds in a distorted fashion in the form of a compromise. Freud always insisted on the 'indestructibility' of the contents of the unconscious. Repressed material not only escapes destruction, it also has a permanent tendency to re-emerge into consciousness. It does so by more or less devious routes... Freud is led to place the emphasis on the fact that the repressed, in order to return, makes use of the same chains of association which have served as the vehicle for repression in the first place... In this context Freud invokes the excuse of the ascetic monk who, while seeking to banish temptation by gazing at an image of the crucifixion, is rewarded by the appearance of a naked woman in the place of the crucified Saviour... 'in and behind the repressing force, what is repressed proves itself victor in the end'."[37]

The spectacle of the priest prepared to murder his son rather than accept him as gay and ill is apparently entirely unremarkable, though its underlying significance is brought out by the son's added comment that "sometimes I think he would like to shoot me whether I had AIDS or not."

In spite of clear recommendations from the National Union of Journalists about the reporting of Aids, and an NUJ booklet of Guidelines for reporting on homosexuality, few journalists themselves seem to have thought very much about the possible consequences of their writings, either for people with Aids and their immediate friends and families, or for the rest of the population. For a long time journalists preferred almost any explanation of the high incidence rate of Aids in central Africa rather than plain old heterosexual sex. Now that the syndrome is so evidently seen not to be confined exclusively to blacks, prostitutes, IV drug-users and gay men, we can only expect yet more frantic retrenchments inside the imaginary fortifications of monogamy, with ever more hysterical denunciations of "the promiscuous". In Britain the Press Council, which is an official watchdog organisation, rejected complaints against the *Sun* for publishing the trigger-happy vicar story. Terry Sanderson of *Gay Times* and Anna Durrell of the Campaign for Homosexual Equality (CHE) alleged that the story was likely to create irrational fears about Aids, and to encourage discrimination or violence against people with the disease. The Press Council concluded...

> "that newspapers should avoid presenting stories dealing with medical matters in a way which causes unnecessary alarm, distress or suffering. In this case the *Sun* chose a dramatic way to focus attention on the danger of Aids. Its article was not presented as medical opinion offered by the paper or as a report of medical opinion, but as a report of the strong views held by a clergyman who had already published similar comments in his parish magazine. The Department of Health and Social Security has agreed that the article did not contain medical inaccuracies, and the Press Council does not find it was likely to provoke discriminatory action against people with Aids. The complaints against the *Sun* are rejected."[38]

This hardly inspires one to trust any institutional control over the "vessels and vassals of power", as Alfred Kazin has described reporters and photographers, who are "never afraid to move in on the moribund and the helpless".[39] A letter from Sally Gilbert, the Equality Officer of the NUJ, to the editor of the *Sun* received the terse reply that...

> "the NUJ's views on Aids in general are of no interest to the *Sun* and have no bearing on our decisions on what to publish".[40]

Journalist Nicholas de Jongh has concluded that "newspapers will continue to write and publish what they choose to until they are made to feel ashamed".[41]

I am less convinced, however, that it is possible to "shame" either journalists or newspaper editors, since irrational stigmatisation is understood by them as professional practice. In any case, newspapers can never be shamed by those whom they so demonstrably hold in both tacit and explicit contempt. This can only remain the case as long as the "queers" are understood as "the moribund and the helpless". An aggressive and unambiguous campaign against homophobic reporting is clearly needed, with direct action when necessary against individual publications. For one unrecognised by-product of such journalism is the steady anger and hostility which it accumulates in those whom it so casually victimises and abuses. It is to newspaper readers that we must turn, offering them publications which will better cater for the diverse needs of a society which the British press seems able only to denounce or to ignore in Canute-like fashion. In this way we can all contribute to the further decline of an industry which is so profoundly anti-democratic and anachronistic, ever more desperately flogging a Victorian moralism which only lives on – to borrow an image from Evelyn Waugh – like a watch still ticking on the wrist of a dead man.

Chapter Six

Aids on television

The reality of Aids is probably no closer to most of the population than the character in Woody Allen's film *Hannah And Her Sisters*, who observes sadly that her dental hygienist now wears rubber gloves because so many of his clients are gay. The underplaying of the line carries a sharp resonance of loss and regret condensed in the tiny incident – a recognition of what is going on, and to whom. Although Aids is not mentioned, this is the only example of which I am aware in mainstream culture of Aids "coming home" as a reality for gay men, who are not simultaneously regarded as if they were creatures from another planet. A recent survey of the British media found that although "it is estimated that at least ten per cent of the population is lesbian or gay", representations "of lesbians and gay men took up 1.85 per cent of television actuality broadcasting time and 0.93 per cent of radio actuality time".[1] Unfortunately, the *London Media Project* which organised the survey, framed its findings in terms of a straightforward distinction between "negative" and "positive" images, with an in-built tendency to think of them as either false or true, as if there were some single "truth" of sexuality which could somehow be broadcast directly across the whole structure of the mass media. Nonetheless, these statistics speak for themselves to a large extent, and behind them lies a series of assumptions about audiences which dominate British and American network broadcasting.

I have argued that homosexuality is constructed as an exemplary and admonitory sign of Otherness in the press, in order to unite sexual and national identifications amongst readers over and above all divisions and distinctions of class, race and gender. Given the close relations between the press and broadcasting, it is not surprising that a similar situation obtains in both television and radio, although the latter, with its stronger commitment to regionalism, is more able to admit lesbians and gay men to the airwaves. We should, however, note that sexuality is subject to a curious double-bind in relation to television, which is regarded as private at the point of viewing, but public in its duties and responsibilities. Unlike newspapers, which strenuously maintain their independence from the state (even and especially when they are supporting the economic and political status quo), television has, since its invention, been understood to require official regulation, especially in relation to questions of obscenity and indecency. The BBC was founded in the 1930s on an assumption "of cultural homogeneity: not that everybody was the same, but that culture was single and undifferentiated".[2] The zoning of programmes at "special interest" groups has maintained this central fiction of a unified national audience, and subsequent legislation has sustained a "concensus" orientation which categorically excludes homosexuality from projections about actual audiences. Thus the Television Act of 1953, which permitted the establishment of commercial broadcasting in the UK, was far more stringent than existing laws about indecency, just as legislation about video in the 1980s has led to greater control than ever over home viewing. The home emerges as a site of great moral danger, with the focus of attention fixed firmly on the possibility of children watching adult programmes. In this context "adult" means sexually explicit, and the result has been a widespread tendency to infantilise the entire notion of the viewing public by preventing the broadcasting of anything which might seem to acknowledge and stimulate childhood sexuality.

The organisation and working practices of television and radio are thus drawn from a reservoir of concerns and categories which in turn derive from a drastically over-simplified estimation of who the television audience is. Any minority which cannot be easily submerged within the flow of television production values will be seen as a "problem", quite independently of its actual social position and experience. Hence the general tendency for lesbians and gay men to find their lives contained within the format of "current affairs" programmes, which are closely subject to direct regulation, and have to maintain strict criteria of "balance". Thus every image of homosexuality is read as a polemic "on behalf of" lesbians or gay men, requiring an answer of some kind, generally in the familiar form of homophobic commentators who are supposed to reassure the "general public". It was this context which guaranteed the failure of London Weekend Television's two series of *Gay Life* magazine programmes in 1980 and 1981, which included an appearance by the veteran anti-gay "clean up television" campaigner Mary Whitehouse to signify the "impartiality" of LWT's Current Affairs Department. As Mandy Merck reflected in *Gay Left* No. 10:

> "If television is not a unified expression of a conspiratorial bourgeois patriarchy, different companies, genres and programmes are nonetheless affected by factors such as legal requirements, stylistic conventions, projected audience reactions, and professional ethics. These factors structure

'the field in which individuals compete to be heard' so subtly
that the programme makers are often the last to recognise
them".[3]

Thus the working practices of the television industry ensure that
lesbians and gay men only emerge into the family living room as
subjects of scandal, humour or humanist pathos. Coded so variously,
according to the requirements of the different genres of television
production, we can see that different types of programme produce
different "knowledges" of homosexuality, and by extension, of
Aids. The most "successful" programme about homosexuality in
recent years was undoubtedly *The Naked Civil Servant*, but its success
lay precisely in the degree to which the central character was
constructed within a discourse of "queerness", which enabled it to
sustain very traditional ideas about gender and sexuality. Much more
interesting is the introduction of gay characters to contemporary
soap operas such as *Brookside*, where a younger son is met by direct
hostility from his father, whilst his fictional mother invited all the
neighbours round to an outdoors barbecue in order to prevent their
seeing a television programme in which the son was due to appear.
Another strand of the plot showed the family's housekeeper resigning
in great anger because she hadn't been told that the son was gay –
assuming that she was at risk of catching Aids from cleaning the
bathroom. The plot thickens...

Such an example of television actually dramatising the exclusion
of gay men from the social consensus, which in this example is
equated with a housing estate near Liverpool where the soap is based,
is, however, far from typical. A recent episode of the current
affairs/chat show hybrid *Where There's Life*, introduced by Dr
Miriam Stoppard, raised problems which are intrinsic to television's
programming and mode of address.[4] Shown in the early evening, in
family viewing time, it dealt with the "issue" of gay teenagers. The
format of the show includes an invited studio audience, ready-made
film inserts, and in this instance a group of young lesbians and gay
men with their mothers. One mother said she was "so relieved to find
it wasn't something dreadful that had happened", to which Miriam
Stoppard replied "I think a lot of parents in this area find the sexual
side very difficult," which was promptly batted straight back at her
by the mother with the statement that

"all parents have difficulties coming to terms with the fact
that their sons and daughters are independent people, and
part of their developing a sexuality is part of their developing
independence."

In this way the mother smartly and effectively demolished Dr Stoppard's double standard about heterosexual and homosexual children. We were then introduced to Frances and her son Steve. "Steven, how old were you when you first felt that you might be gay?" asked Dr Stoppard, significantly not asking him in direct terms how old he was when he realised he *was* gay. Steve replied that he was nine. "At *nine*?" came the reply, with a tone of barely concealed astonishment and disbelief, as if he had just confessed to having robbed a bank. Steven then went on to talk about his early awareness of sexual difference, and his growing self-awareness at about the age of eleven. Dr Stoppard then turned to his mother: "Did you actually say to him 'you're too young to know this, you can't know this'?" and was again rebuffed with a plain "No. I didn't think he was too young to know it," once more rejecting the implicit meaning behind the question. Had he told her that he'd been sexually molested, doubts about the age factor would undoubtedly not have been invoked.

Steven then described a letter from his father which had argued that sex is about having babies, at which point Dr Stoppard interrupted him: "In the end though, sex *is* about procreation isn't it? In a biological sense we have to keep the race going," and, as if answering her own question, adding "that's true". Steven, however, denied her argument, pointing out that sex is as much about the release of tension as about anything else. Whether Dr Stoppard was stating her own views or speaking "on behalf" of her imagined audience at home, she nonetheless offered a most extraordinarily naive attitude towards sex, and I should add that her public come-uppance was a considerable pleasure to behold. We then heard from another mother, this time of a lesbian called Linda: "Here was my daughter. I was not going to give her up . . . she was my child. I loved her, so I had to adapt." Asked if she felt "a sense of loss or bereavement" she yet again exposed the assumption behind the question: "No. I sense I've gained something," and Linda proceeded to describe how coming out had brought her much closer to the rest of her family. This was too much for Dr Stoppard, who turned to camera with the final words: "So, if this does happen in your family, try and remember that it always is possible to come to terms with it in the end," closing down the discussion as if it hadn't happened, returning her audience unhesitatingly to an alignment of homosexuality with the status of "problem" and embarrassment. Would she have found it so difficult to accept a boy "confessing" to the realisation of heterosexuality at the age of nine? Would she expect a parent to doubt a child's self-knowledge about heterosexuality at the age of eleven? I think not, and such questions betray a much wider tendency to frame all discussion of homosexuality within the terms and values of a consensus which is legislative and ideological rather than apparent from the position of actual television spectators across the social and sexual spectrum. Although Aids was not mentioned in the programme, this is also the framework from which television thinks the subject in the first place.

In February, 1985, *Weekend World* asked *"The AIDS Question"*. Or rather, several questions, including "What Is The Source?", "How Many Succumb?" and so on, the answers to which provided the programme with its format. Each question was framed as a caption, above a colour photograph of an anonymous person with Aids whose face had been badly disfigured, which reappeared throughout the programme. The presenter, Brian Walden, guided us through the issues as perceived for a popular but serious Sunday programme. Early on a clear distinction was usefully made between HIV infection and Aids by Richard Tedder, a medical virologist at London's Middlesex Hospital, who also talked of "Aids sufferers" rather than "victims". David Miller, a clinical psychologist at St Mary's, Paddington, described sexually "active" gay men as being at particular risk, adding that gay men are especially "mobile" so that "the virus tends to be spread more widely than it might otherwise be". This was not, I think, a version of an all-homosexual-men-are-middle-class argument. Rather, it relates to the fact that many gay men have visited the United States in recent years. What it elides, however, is the reason why we went there in such numbers in the first place, which can only be explained in relation to the dismal experience of growing up gay and British, without the kind of affirmative gay culture which made New York and San Francisco into places of pilgrimage and inspiration throughout the 1970s. Walden, however, moved straight in to claim that

> "gay men now have an interest in sharply reducing the number of their sexual partners. They should also take great care when choosing them. Indeed, the only really safe course for gay men is to stick to one partner or to avoid oral and anal sex completely."

This is the litany which runs on and on through television Aids commentary and, quite apart from the most peculiar assumption that we don't in any case "take great care when choosing" with whom we have sex, it equates monogamy with safety in a highly irresponsible manner. What matters is what you *do* sexually, not with how many people.

The programme also explained that there is a risk from bisexual men having sex with gay men and passing the virus on to heterosexual women. In this respect the commentary spelled out what had been implied in a diagram shown on an earlier *Weekend World* which was also about Aids. Here gay men had been pictured as a line of boogy-ing disco dancers at the bottom of the image, above whom was positioned the familiar figure of the family – mum and dad and two small children. In between these two distinct groups two single figures were posed, a prostitute and a bi-sexual, the former female, the latter male. The ideological significance of such diagrams is important to grasp. In the first place we are invited to imagine some absolute divide between the two domains of "gay life" and "the family", as if gay men grew up, were educated, worked and lived our lives in total isolation from the rest of society. Second, we are to think of the bi-sexual as an "active" penetrative male, who can carry the HIV virus up from the infernal domain of Discoland and into the very bosom of the nuclear family. Third, the prostitute appears in her familiar ideological apparel as Fallen Eve, the contaminated vessel, literally a *femme fatale*. But what of female bi-sexuality? What of male prostitution? And, above all, what of the father/husband or wife/mother, moving unseen across the picture to consort with these deadly bedfellows? What is at stake here is the mystifying and mischievous pattern of associations which makes male equal active, and female equal passive. This is the same system of slippages which casts homo-sexuality as a species of gender-confusion rather than a fluctuating field of sexual desires and behaviour.

According to Walden, "bisexuality is more widespread than is sometimes appreciated", and "wives and girl friends might find themselves at risk". The point here is that if he is correct, then a large parcel of blame should be laid at the feet of a media industry which has consistently refused to acknowledge the sexual diversity of its actual spectators, preferring to cater for the amazing fiction of a uniformly and unproblematically heterosexual general public. But for Walden this merely leads on to "the most difficult question Aids poses. Will the disease stay mainly confined to a small number of specific groups" (where, presumably, he thinks it will eventually burn itself out – together with perhaps twenty million gay men in Europe alone) "or will it leak out into the rest of the population to pose a general threat?" There are reasons, he claimed, "for hoping that leakage will be very limited". These include the supposed physio-logical weakness of the rectum, compared to the vagina, a comparison frequently made in such documentary contexts, regard-less of the fact that vaginal fluid and semen are equally infectious, and that blood contact with either can and does take place as frequently during vaginal as anal intercourse. At this point Robin McKie, whom we have met before as science correspondent for the *Observer*, is brought on stage to talk about the threat of "leakage" to "the heterosexual community", whatever that might be, concluding that indeed the epidemic will tail off only when it has run out of "high-risk" victims, a prospect the enormity of which seems not to concern him. So, according to Walden, "except for those who are male homosexuals, there's a limit to what we can do as individuals. But on a major issue of public health we can look to the government to act." In other words, it is up to gay men to sort themselves out, whilst government must intervene to protect everybody else. In just this way gay men are tacitly yet inexorably positioned somewhere quite outside the social formation, and television's range of interest.

Fortunately, at this point Professor Michael Adler reminded us that Aids is "a major public health problem for those who are suffering from it", thus putting gay people with Aids, and gay men as a whole, back into place as part of "the public". But he is no more heard than Miriam Stoppard heard the gay teenagers talking about their childhoods, for he was immediately followed by Robin McKie cheerfully stating his opinion that "there would be a lot of political advantage for the government in taking a tough line with the gay community over the question of Aids", with compulsory screenings, monitoring, and so on. Fortunately, however, he was at least to some extent playing devil's advocate, since he went on to spell out the larger danger that Aids would then be forced "underground", as Terry Webb from *Gay Switchboard* had argued earlier in the programme. Nor would such an approach help or encourage anyone to seek medical advice, or consider taking an HIV test in the absence of medical confidentiality. Peter West, a health economist from the University of Aberdeen, then argued against a state-run counselling service on the grounds of expense – in spite of the fact that on the latest estimates it costs on average nearly £7,000 to treat people with Aids from the initial diagnosis to death.[5] And just for good measure he added that such support for "AIDS victims" might be "difficult" because "people might object". That such objections are comparable only to objections made against helping Japanese victims of the bombings of Hiroshima and Nagasaki in 1945 do not occur to Mr West.

Brian Walden then proceeded to interview Mr John Patton, the Minister handling Aids policy at government level. After much mutual congratulation and evasion Patton stated that this "isn't a problem where one can just throw money at the problem and make it go away", echoing a major rhetorical trope of Thatcherite monetarist thought – although this is precisely a problem which will *only* go away if money is thrown at it, and lots of it. Patton described the then reported number of cases of Aids in the UK as "very small": the figure mentioned was 118. One cannot help asking whose standards define 118 fatalities in such a way, regardless of the fact that he was being culpably disingenuous about statistics, knowing full well the epidemiological projections for the spread of the syndrome. He did speak directly against "punitive" government action however, as if government under-funding, and its total failure to provide an adequate information scheme, were not effectively punitive in themselves. The minister ended by refusing to answer questions about "risk", referring back to "experts" like Robin McKie whom he warmly, and frighteningly, congratulated, adding finally that he would be quite prepared to meet an "AIDS victim", share a glass with him, shake hands, and sit next to him to be interviewed.

This gauntlet was promptly picked up by Thames Television, who stage-managed just such a meeting a few weeks later in *AIDS – The Victims*. Throughout the programme a discourse of "Aids victims" was maintained, from the opening announcement that

> "tonight *TV Eye* talks to those with the killer disease Aids. One of the victims is in hospital, the other is at home. Both are in their mid thirties and homosexual. They tell what it's like learning to live under sentence of death, and ask will society learn to live with them too."

This introduction also served to disguise the actual production of the programme, offering a "reality" which is always, as Stuart Hall points out, an illusion:

> " – the 'naturalistic illusion' – since the combination of verbal and visual discourse which produces this effect of 'reality' requires the most skilful and elaborate procedures of coding: mounting, linking and stitching elements together, working them into a system of narration or exposition which 'makes sense'".[6]

One man with Aids was questioned with considerable insensitivity, for instance when asked by reporter Peter Prendergast if he was "frightened" or "depressed". Fortunately Dr Anthony Pinching was at hand to talk down casual contact scaremongering, which he did in his customary efficient way, reinforcing the point that Aids "is not a very infectious disease". Asked if there is "a cure for Aids" he patiently explained the distinction between damage to one's immune system, and individual opportunistic infections which result from that damage, and are treated accordingly.

Prendergast, however, registered nothing of this, suffering from a common case of Aids-commentator's amnesia, and merely blundered straight on to describe how "John got Aids through homosexual contact in America. It is the promiscuous nature of parts of the gay community which has helped spread the disease across the world". Not content with reading Aids as a product of sexual activity as such, he conjured up a vision of world-wide "promiscuity" at the same time as he implicitly distinguished between "good" gays (i.e., non-promiscuous, like "us", the television audience and its reporter) and "bad" gays, who have lots of disgusting sex and get Aids. As we have however already seen, being "good" in these terms has little to do with risk of HIV infection. Another gay man stated explicitly in the same programme that you can't blame yourself for contracting a virus which you didn't know existed, particularly when its asympto-matic incubation period may have been anything up to five years. He described himself as "a relatively well-adjusted gay person, and yes I have sex with other people", adding that he had not had sex with anyone else in the past fifteen or so months. The scene then changed to show him writing his diary, as the voice-over loftily claimed that "at least Bill, as he himself admits, knew the risk and took his chances". In fact he had said nothing of the kind, but Prendergast is only interested in what anybody actually says as long as it supports his own agenda, which in this case required the establishment of a firm distinction between "innocent" and "guilty" victims.

The epidemic was then traced back to central Africa by Dr Jonathan Weaver, described as an "Aids expert", who was filmed in an office with a slide of a blood sample enlargement projected on the wall behind him as a sign of medical "authority". Having discussed the heterosexual context of Aids in Africa, Weaver went on to say that "one gay man acquiring the virus, perhaps even sexually acquiring the virus in Zaire, could have brought this back to New York City in the late Seventies, and the whole epidemic of Aids could have stemmed from that". Thus alignment with homosexuality is made to over-ride the fact that, like any other virus, it conspicuously fails to recognise sexual difference of any kind. It also reinforced the programme's underlying project, announced clearly over a shot of a middle-aged woman seated in a small sitting room, who stood in for all the "other groups of people whose lifestyle is a world apart, but who've also been caught up in the same tragedy". The intended meaning is clear enough, but it is slipped into the unspoken assumption that the woman in question is not "promiscuous", and therefore not to blame. This was brought home as she described the slow death of her haemophiliac husband from Aids.

The gay man with Aids *was* allowed to criticise the reporting of Aids in the press, and clippings from newspapers were shown at the beginning of the programme, another familiar device in television coverage, suggesting as it were that "we" in television are not like "them" in the gutter press. It should already be clear, however, that the agenda of Aids reporting crosses over between different media, even if they resort to different means to make their common points. The inclusion of David Miller from St Mary's, Paddington, who also attacked press coverage, seemed yet another element edited in to disavow the massive homophobia of the *TV Eye* project. The programme ended with its little "scoop", the meeting between the minister and the gay man with Aids, who were shown very briefly together before the voice-over cut them off: "the minister and the Aids victim – a public show of confidence in a world of private uncertainty". The imaginary audience was clearly intended to line up with John Patten at this point, but I wonder how many other viewers took it for granted that any minister serving under Mrs Thatcher is seriously dangerous, unlike the man with Aids.

The use of this "victim" was far from isolated and *The London Programme*, later in 1985, had little difficulty finding people who could be edited in such a way as to embody homophobic fantasy. Opening with a set-up newspaper hoarding which read "AIDS: New London Victim", the voice-over asked, "Will the capital's gays be able to adapt to protect themselves?", followed by a sequence of headlines from the tabloid press, and the statement that most "of Britain's AIDS victims are homosexuals from London, and now the government is taking action to control the disease". The entire style and look of *The London Programme* is tabloid, and exemplifies the way in which television and the press huddle together and feed off one another in an endless loop of commentary, reviews and so on. So, in the best tradition of the *Sun*, *The London Programme* sent out an intrepid reporter to conduct random interviews, asking people in the street what they thought Aids is. In fact there was a significantly high level of informed response, which was presumably somewhat inconvenient to the programme makers' requirements, to the extent that the voice-over felt obliged to cap the sequence with a bald and vacuous claim that "the public mind" sees Aids as "a gay disease". This was followed by "quickie" interviews with a professional embalmer and a tattooist, both of whom were there to say collectively that they would no longer embalm or tattoo gay men, though one wonders just how they decide their clients' sexuality. The programme's approach effortlessly trivialised the real difficulties experienced by people with Aids, in relation to dental care for example, by setting up such false problems. The voice-over repeated that "Aids is not exclusively homosexual", but this sounded suspiciously like more disavowal, given the reiterated and completely spurious assumption that any virus is in any sense attracted by nature to any particular sexuality. The scene then shifted to the large London gay club, *Heaven*, with floor level shots constructing the dancing men as towering monstrous figures, etched in flickering lights. London was described as "tolerant", and this supposedly explains the existence of a flourishing gay scene. Needless to say, the logic of this observation was not carried back to questions of why gay men are so frequently forced to leave smaller towns and cities for no other reason than their sexuality. The voice-over went on to argue that gay men, as the social group which is most at risk from Aids, have it in their power to prevent its spread.

At this point an extract from the 1981 *Gay Life* series was spliced into the programme. Two older men were seen talking about the London gay scene of the 1930s, whilst the Gay Liberation movement was read as a response to the liberalisation of Wolfenden Strategy, rather than its failure. The commentary made the point that "homosexuals became gays" but seemed unable to make anything of the distinction which it had tentatively established. An old clip of the gay historian and activist Jeffrey Weeks was inserted to make the point that Gay Liberation was primarily about sex, and the commentary moved on to "explain" how the new clubs and social facilities of the 1970s had made sex much more easily available, thus leading, apparently, to an emphasis on quick relationships. The voice-over then talked of the "extreme promiscuity" of the American gay scene, suggesting a direct and uncomplicated relationship between casual sex and Aids. Some safe sex advice was offered from The Terrence Higgins Trust and Julian Meldrum, followed by an interview with a gay couple, sitting on a park bench, one of whom described their relationship as a "man-and-wife" marriage, with "no extra-marital affairs". But, continued the voice-over, "for many London gays" this "would not be acceptable".

After a quick burst of statistics we were returned to a gay bar in South London, where one young gay man explained that he had no family or lover, so changing his sex life would be difficult. He telephoned the television studios some days later to inform them that he had just tested positive to HIV, and was re-interviewed, as if to cement the immediate connection between gay sex and Aids. The voice-over intoned self-righteously that "if one section of the gay community doesn't adapt, more Aids deaths seem probable. So London will have to brace itself for a greater increase in Aids infections". As we know, there is simply no such thing as an "Aids infection". That did not worry London Weekend Television, however, since the project behind this programme was clearly to isolate and establish the notion that there is a group of "irresponsible" gay men at large, deliberately refusing to change their ways, in spite of everything a homophobic press and broadcast media has screamed at them. The voice-over attempted at this point to make a distinction between those "reluctant" to change their sexual behaviour, conceived numerically, and those who are "unable", thus mobilising a type of "will" versus "instinct" approach to safe sex. Aids publicity was also described as a possible pretext for renewed hostility to gay men, but this was hardly convincing since such hostility has in any case never gone away. It was left to Jeffrey Weeks to argue that "in modern society homosexuals are partially tolerated but homosexuality still isn't". This is revealed in "what's happened over the last few months", and is based on "deep levels of anxiety and fear about homosexuality in a wider society... a very delicate situation" in which it is only too easy for the "moral right to exploit the situation and to begin a crusade against homosexuality as such". This is perilously close to what *The London Programme* managed to achieve.

The gay Labour MP Chris Smith also warned against the danger of hysteria and over-reaction, and LWT obliged with the example of a cartoon in the *Sun* which showed Smith seated alone in the House of Commons, shunned by his colleagues. Peter Tatchell, the Labour politician and writer, talked about the verbal and physical abuse he had endured when standing as a parliamentary candidate at the last general election but, again, whatever he might have had to say was undermined by the programme's glib description of him as "another confessed homosexual". He was followed by an arbitrary interview with a young gay man who had been sacked from his job because he was gay, before we cut back again to the "married" gay couple, whose marital status was inscribed in the fact that one spoke for both, whilst his friend merely nodded assent. "They" described how they had been ordered out of their local Working Men's Club without so much as finishing their drinks, although I wondered what on earth they were doing there in the first place. The voice-over was however permitted to ramble on witlessly about "the first stirrings of social intolerance" which, in the context of a programme ostensibly about Aids, was a singularly banal observation. The programme ended with the identification of two "problems", firstly the "refusal" to change sexual "habits" on the part of some gay men and, secondly, the possible infection of heterosexuals. The final credit sequence rolled up over a still photograph of the interior of an East London Leather bar, resonating with connotations of sexuality, and a last depressing comment about the absence of any cure and the long time-factor involved in research, as if to say "time's up" on gay sex.

All of this was a far cry from an extended item on Aids in the context of British trade unionism, shown later in 1985 on Channel Four's *Union World*, which organised its discussion in relation to a speaker at the 1985 Labour Party Annual Conference who had publicly equated Aids with "unnatural acts". A series of interviews examined individual cases of job discrimination, and then turned to trade union representatives from a number of different industrial sectors. It was, for example, explained by a speaker from the National Union of Public Employees nurses' group that blood is frequently an occupational hazard for hospital workers, and that singling out the HIV virus was absurd. Despite bad news from the British Aids charity The Terrence Higgins Trust about the refusal of trades unions to co-operate with their information programme, David Miller, a clinical psychologist from St Mary's, Paddington, rounded up by stressing the injustices and cruelty involved in discrimination against people who already have to live with the day to day anxiety of having tested positive.

Whilst British television documentary practice is not necessarily caught in the same trap of "impartial" production values as Current Affairs, it is, however, closely caught up with strong notions of "prestige", especially given its great expense in relation to other forms of television production. Thus the calculation of potential sales to overseas networks has tended to work against innovation and risk taking as perceived by production teams and companies alike. Documentary television is also widely regarded as the "flagship" genre of individual competing networks, whilst the portentous legacy of the British documentary film movement works further to inhibit and ossify its working practices. In this respect there are few more comfortably respectable fronts for virulent homophobia than the notion of scientific objectivity. For a recent BBC *Horizon* team the combination of virology, immunology, epidemiology and homo-sexuality proved irresistible. *AIDS: A Strange and Deadly Virus*[7] opened with a car driving at night into what appeared to be a heavily guarded military site, which indeed it was, as the voice-over informed us after a good dose of grotesquely inappropriate, eerie sci-fi "suspense" music:

> "US Army Fort Dietrich, once renowned for biological warfare experiments; today more Aids virus is produced here than anywhere else in the world".

Our old friend the "Aids virus" alerts us instantly, like a smoke detector, to the presence of grave ideological danger ahead... We follow elaborate security measures into the laboratories, positioned behind the creeping, twisting camera like children playing peek-a-boo, as the doom-laden voice informs us that "over the last three or four years we have seen every one of our worst predictions confirmed". Quite who "we" are in this scenario is not made clear, though it immediately serves to unite "us", the television audience, with "them", the programme makers.

The structure and behaviour of the virus was explained very clearly with recourse to elaborate and very effective computer graphics which, after a brief introduction to Dr Robert Gallo of the US National Cancer Institute, led on to the social setting of the syndrome. We met a young newlywed couple, Bruce and Bobbie, who had been a nurse until she contracted Aids after being infected by the virus from a blood transfusion. Then, after a lengthy section dealing with a psychological study of people exposed to the virus, we were told that "over fifty per cent of Aids patients may ultimately become demented". In this context "may" is hardly a helpful word, but it enhanced the general fatalism of the scientific commentary. Thus the figure of "tens of thousands dying" was dutifully accompanied by more doom-laden suspense music, which neatly carried over the accumulating associations of horror and dread to descriptions of "homosexual spread" in Brazil and elsewhere.

An unidentified black delegate to a conference in Brussels was introduced next to pursue this line of thought, saying his piece about newly urbanised and displaced young men in central Africa who apparently "fall prey to these practices", with the implication that Aids arrived in Uganda and Zaire and elsewhere as the direct result of white gay tourists having sex with Africans, who are thus presented as yet another "vulnerable" group. And how convenient for the makers of the programme to find a black man to articulate the familiar infantilising discourse of "the natives". Prostitutes were dealt with in a similar fashion, as we saw something of the work of *Project Aware*, a women's group which sets out to inform other women about Aids. This involved nocturnal street patrols, which certainly looked extremely like nineteenth-century social purity campaigners out to "save" fallen women, an impression reinforced by two highly questionable interviews, one with a "specimen" prostitute describing her work in the sex industry, the other with a young punkish woman framed as "promiscuous", though in fact she talked very sensibly about birth control methods. But that was hardly the point, for she was only there to personify a "risk" group, and to serve as an admonitory prelude to the uniquely disgusting contribution from Professor Opendra Narayan of the Johns Hopkins Medical School.

Seated at his desk in front of a large Mannerist painting of semi-naked men, Narayan proceeded to divide up gay men into the "active" and the "passive", describing the rectum as an "unhygienic environment" which tears and bleeds easily. According to Narayan, whose background lies in veterinary medicine,

> "the active sexual partner injects infected semen into the anus of the passive partner ... These people have sex twenty

to thirty times a night . . . A man comes along and goes from anus to anus and in a single night will act as a mosquito transferring infected cells on his penis. When this is practised for a year, with a man having three thousand sexual intercourses, one can readily understand this massive epidemic that is currently upon us."

Given that Narayan prefers a theory of infection by direct cell to cell transfer, this is fairly breathtakingly inconsistent, since it is only by the wildest flight of fantasy that any man could be thought capable of ten, let alone thirty separate orgasms, each with different partners, every night. But this is the commonsense of homophobia to which doctors, given the extreme narrowness of their education and social experience, as well as their notoriously conservative professional practices, are especially prone. It is just this type of voice which so increases the anxiety of gay men in relation to the medical profession.

Bobbie, the heterosexual woman with Aids, talked of the bad treatment which she had received as an ex-nurse from other working nurses, raising the issue of how they might deal with the "other patients there", in other words the "guilty" patients. A Japanese scientist named "Mitch to his friends" described his research work, and was promptly referred to as Mitch, on the assumption that we are his "friends", with shots of the virus stored in laboratory conditions, with workers in masks and gowns and plastic bags over their heads. Such shots casually reinforce a totally spurious picture of Aids as a syndrome requiring extraordinary precautionary measures. The fascination of Aids documentary makers with the sight of needles in arms, intravenous drips, animal experiments and so on, crosses almost every programme on the subject, thus amplifying a general sense of physical horror about treatment which is most unhelpful. The programme ended with the work of a British epidemiologist in San Francisco, where we are told that more than fifty per cent of gay men are HIV positive, and where "a determined effort has been made to educate people". Nonetheless,

> "the verdict on whether sexual restraint actually makes a difference is in the blood of Andrew Moss' subjects . . . While the victims live on in the hope of a cure, and those at risk a vaccine, medical science is still struggling to come up with an answer to Aids".

Thus gay people with Aids are viewed as either good, obedient subjects, accepting medical authority unquestioningly, or as bad subjects, "refusing" this authority, a distinction which is all the more difficult for people with Aids in America because of the wide range of starkly conflicting opinions on offer to them from different doctors, that is, if they can afford to go to doctors in the first place. The final scene showed a Christmas party in a San Francisco Aids clinic, with women and men singing, and two men clinging together weeping, cutting away to Bobbie and her husband ice-skating, with a final word from Dr Gallo, thus closing on the note of firm medical authority which had run through the entire programme.

Similar problems affect fictionalised depictions of the epidemic. Thus at the pre-production state of NBC's *An Early Frost*,

> "the real issue of concern to the network's broadcast standards department was not so much the presentation of Aids as the treatment of homosexuality. According to one source close to the production, the NBC censor said to the producer, 'I thought we were doing a film about Aids, not about homosexuality.' And the producer said to him, 'What planet have you been living on?' If this were a heterosexual Aids movie, there would have been no problems at all. But the network is terrified of doing anything that might seem to be condoning homosexuality. The grandmother can't say to her grandson, 'I think your boyfriend is nice,' because that might seem to be an endorsement of homosexuality. Those were the things that were constantly being changed".[8]

It is precisely this level of institutional censorship which guarantees a constant muting effect throughout the representation of Aids on television, rationalised as "professionalism", and justified in commercial terms of ratings.

An Early Frost showed all the evidence of being just such a compromise formation, manufactured from the conflicting wishes of the script-writers and the network, aligning itself with its "responsibilities" to "the public". Thus the story of one young New York gay man, Michael Pierson, who contracts Aids, was narrated half-way between the conventions of terminal illness romance films like *Dark Victory* or *Love Story*, and the "new" Hollywood gay populism of *Making Love* and *Brothers*.[9] Michael's situation is viewed from the locus of his family, and the film's central theme is the reconciliation of father to son, with the threat of death as the only way his father can accept Michael's being gay. This is, in fact, an updated "coming out" story, with Aids as little more than a narrative device. Darrel Yates Rist has argued that

> "while no-one expects NBC to show the Pierson boy tonguing on the television screen, a little hugging, maybe a few tears – *something* in their private moments together would have helped validate their love, or dramatise that

> these two guys are more than room-mates, more than best friends who fuck off screen".[10]

Yet this somehow misses the point that beneath the family romance there is another film altogether, about a gay man who is so crippled by guilt that he refers to his lover of two years as "a neighbour" to his family. Throughout the film there is an infuriating ambiguity of purpose, so that when Michael's pregnant sister, who has refused to come anywhere near him as he convalesces from an early opportunistic infection, yells at her mother "What would *you* have done?" there is simply no reply. We are supposed to side with Michael *and* his sister, *and* his tiresome macho father. The closing shot is thus all the more unfortunate since it shows a "family album" picture of the Pierson family, united, after Michael's death – but of course without his boy friend. A traumatic episode is over. The family closes ranks, with the problem son conveniently dispatched, and life getting back to normal...

Arthur Bressan Jr's *Buddies*[11] demonstrates that drama can "tell a good story while teaching a number of facts".[12] The titles go up over an ominous and seemingly interminable computer print-out of names, names which we assume to be of people with Aids. Here the story concerns Robert, a young gay man from San Francisco who is in hospital in New York, and David, his "buddy" from a gay centre, who befriends him. Robert is constructed as a fairly typical gay man of the Gay Liberation period, intensely aware of the politics of sexuality, whilst David is shown as a rather complacent Yuppie. In fact it is almost inconceivable (one hopes) that someone as ignorant about Aids should ever be allowed near Robert or, for that matter, that he would ever have been aware of the mere existence of a gay centre, let alone have got involved in such a project. Robert had been thrown out of his home by his parents when he told them he was gay. David, on the contrary, has an impossibly supportive mother, whose phone calls punctuate the entire narrative. At the outset David judges Robert's life as wasted by his commitment to gay politics, and a seven year "open" relationship which he reads as a total failure. Asked what he'd do if he could have a single day out of hospital and be "well", Robert replies that he'd fly to Washington and march up and down in front of the White House with a banner protesting against the under-funding of hospital and support care for people with Aids, and then fly back to his old boy friend Edward and fuck his brains out. Gradually David comes to understand the culture which Robert is coming from, a culture which he, in his luxurious apartment with a monogamous relationship and a "Designer everything" mentality, has never come across. He realises slowly that the privacy which he so jealously cherishes only came about as a result of the struggles of people like Robert and Edward. His new understanding is signified in a beautiful scene where he holds Robert in his arms whilst he jerks off, looking at a photograph of Edward. David is finally persuaded to give a newspaper interview about his work as a buddy since, as Robert says, it might help someone somewhere to come to a better attitude towards the epidemic. But, when he takes the paper into the hospital, he finds that Robert has died, suddenly and unexpectedly. The film ends with a shot of David, walking up and down outside the White House amongst the crowds of indifferent tourists, holding up a banner with Robert's words on it. The film thus addresses precisely the issue of the re-homosexualisation of gay culture which Aids has opened up. It suggests a level of personal integrity, and the sheer complexity of the situation in which people with Aids find themselves, that has not been touched upon in any of the documentaries shown on British television to date.

Of these, the most recent was also the most obnoxious. *AIDS is a four-letter word*[13] opened with a shot of crowds outside London's Albery Theatre, where Larry Kramer's play *The Normal Heart* was showing. A male voice-over immediately moved in to warn us that "Aids is no longer a disease which only affects minorities", as if it ever had been. "In 1980 it threatens us all". This hardly needs to be elaborately unpicked: the implication is clear – now that it's not "just" queers and prostitutes, drug addicts and black Africans who are at risk, "we", the "general public", need to protect ourselves, and "we" in television are doing just that. The programme's presenter, Christine Chapman, took precisely this line, arguing that Aids is more than a medical problem, it is also a moral issue, and "our only protection against Aids is radically to alter our sexual behaviour". Aids, she claimed,

> "is a sexually transmitted disease, not the most shattering of statements, but it does explain why we haven't been able to stop a fatal and incurable virus from reaching epidemic proportions – not because we're embarrassed about venereal disease, not because we're too shy to talk about sex, but because from the very start we simply haven't been able to face the moral questions that Aids asks about sexual freedom".

A number of things need to be said at this point. To begin with, Aids is *not* a venereal disease, though this is a necessary connection for Chapman to establish in order to support her conclusions. Secondly, the virus is *not* fatal, although there is as yet no known way of rebuilding the immunological defences of people who go on to develop opportunistic infections. Thirdly, her slip back from the modern discourse of "sexually transmitted diseases" to "venereal disease", with all its baggage of pejorative connotations and shame, is extremely significant, again in the light of what is to follow. Fourthly, Aids as such doesn't ask any questions. People do, and they do so from a variety of motives. Any attempt to speak in the name of any illness is immediately highly suspect. It shows that something is being covered up, that a subtle and suspect ventriloquism is at work.

We then move to a meeting between Paul, a gay man with Aids, and his unnamed doctor. His body, the voice-over explains, "has lost its defence against infection, so his health must be constantly monitored. Any passing bug, harmless to you and me, may now be fatal to Paul" who "knows the odds are stacked against him". This is yet another case of television Aids-commentators' amnesia, since what Paul immediately says loudly and clearly is that he is determined "to live with a capital L ... I'm not going to crawl away and die – I'm going to do everything I can to prolong my life, as long as the quality of my life remains good". Against a marching army of computer graphic humanoids the voice-over continues: "Aids doesn't mind if you're gay or straight" (unlike Ms Chapman) and "is likely to claim more victims as time goes on. What we're seeing is only the tip of the iceberg. Aids is a silent and hidden epidemic". As this programme demonstrates, Aids is anything but a "silent epidemic", even though the volume which it generates is guaranteed to ensure that the day-to-day realities of most people with Aids are certainly very well "hidden" indeed. As for the iceberg, one can only conclude that there is no shortage of Sloane Rangers and Young Fogeys like Ms Chapman, lurking just under the surface of British television, eagerly waiting to follow her "courageous" moral example ...

Professor Robin Weiss, Director of the Institute for Cancer Research, turns up next to air his statistics, saying that

> "somewhere between twenty and one hundred thousand people in this country [the UK] are infected. Many of these will eventually develop Aids. So we know, even if we could stop it spreading from today onwards, that we would still see very many more cases than we've seen to date, and that cannot be prevented".

The voice-over proceeds to suggest that the ratio of people who are antibody positive to those with Aids has been drastically under-estimated, with much reference to the non-existent "Aids virus", and none to any concrete evidence supporting this hypothesis. Weiss then reappears, after a generally aimless discussion of dementia amongst people with Aids, to sketch in a "worst case" scenario, enthusiastically offering an apocalyptic vision of the future, in which seventy per cent of the population of Britain has been infected, and the "remaining" thirty per cent cannot protect themselves since there would be a hopeless shortage of healthy blood donors. The situation of the seventy per cent is, of course, totally disregarded. So Chapman repeats, in the absence of a vaccine let alone a cure, "an epidemic that can't be cured must be contained, but again, everywhere we turn we still can't face up to the moral question that Aids raises about sexual freedom". Clearly "we" are positioned here with the threatened thirty per cent, in the context of a highly inflammatory discourse of "containment", and a seemingly obsessive litany of denial about our supposed inability to "face up" to moral issues. The real problem here is the inability of Christine Chapman to "face up" to any other moral position beyond her own, let alone to any other aspects of Aids – such as the politics of funding, education and support groups, on all of which she maintains a deafening silence.

It is, however, time for another appearance by Professor Weiss, who at least recognises the impracticality of any suggestion that sex should at once be stopped in all its forms. He is therefore thrown back to a less preferable possibility of universal, one hundred per cent sexual monogamy, which again he concedes to be unrealisable, "but it could well prove that the Aids epidemic and the mass deaths that will follow in the wake of the virus" could lead to a change in "our social attitudes, but perhaps change them too late". This kind of voluntarism ties in closely with that of Chapman, both turning round on the point of conscious moral choice supposedly leading to immediate behavioural change. How the will might be mobilised against deeply engrained patterns of desire is not for one moment contemplated. In the rugged world of moralism, the will appears an heroic thing, able to change an identity without internal resistance of any kind, as if sexuality is endlessly open to such expedient correctives. The banality of this vision explains why the programme then shifted its attention to the "problem" of promiscuity, including a discussion from *The Normal Heart*, which was much more complex than Ms Chapman seemed to realise. Nonetheless it was sufficient to lead into the voice-over's assertion that for gay men "any attack on promiscuity was seen as an attack on the right to be gay, and that's still the problem".

This amazing over-simplification hangs on an unstated moral imperative which is implicit in the use of the term promiscuity. Spelled out loud, this insists that monogamy is an intrinsic and absolute good, to be contrasted to the intrinsic and absolute bad of all other kinds of sexual behaviour. Most people, however, do not "choose" monogamy; they "choose" sexual partners, against a wide variety of criteria and circumstances. Promiscuity is in essence a theological concept, deriving from the Christian attitude to the sanctity of marriage as a sacramental act. It is thus inseparable from the institution of Christian marriage and child-raising, as well as the larger patriarchal Judaeo-Christian tradition of patriarchal morality. As a concept it is thus entirely redundant in relation to same-sex relationships, unless the people involved are Christian, and regard themselves as theologically married. It is the exclusive equation of monogamy with morality which privileges enforced fidelity over and above all questions of consent. Commentators like Christine Chapman, who invariably strike brave postures about the need to "face facts", are merely pandering to a fashionable authoritarianism in order to justify their thinly-veiled wish to impose a moral straightjacket on all those who do not share their archaic religious inclinations. We do not, in fact, choose between "promiscuity" and "monogamy", whatever our sexual orientation : we choose between one another, freely and mutually, to the evident horror of those who proceed from an initial disapproval of sexual pleasure as an end in itself.

Hence the tack which Chapman follows in her programme, importing a speaker from The Terrence Higgins Trust to talk, very briefly, about safe sex, only to cut him off mid sentence with the words: "In the end you can't do much, although you can do it with as many people as you like". The flippancy of such an attitude can only be explained in terms of a profound anxiety about numbers of sexual partners, abstracted from social life and regarded in a moral vacuum. For to dismiss safe sex is to dismiss the one, incontrovertible means of defence against the spread of the virus. That Christine Chapman could only bring herself to acknowledge the existence of arguments about safe sex education, but refusing any detailed discussion, should suggest something of her motives throughout this thoroughly emetic programme. A middle-aged woman with Aids spoke next, her face in shadow, but her voice and surroundings coding her as respectable. She described safe sex as

> "extremely difficult to stick to. If one has spent one's entire life being 'good in bed', are you suddenly going to say, 'Oh! I don't do *that*'. So it is difficult . . . I would recommend either celibacy if you are known to be a carrier – it's not much fun. Who wants to stay at home and masturbate when you can have a lovely time with a partner? But I think you owe it to society and yourself . . ."

There was no "or" following on from her "either", which suggests she said something else which didn't fit in with Chapman's project.

Not that what she did say made much sense, since "the lovely time with a partner" sounds quite compatible with safe sex. But it was the magic word "celibacy" which was wanted at that point. Having used it she had fulfilled her purpose.

Martin Weaver from The Terrence Higgins Trust then made a reappearance, putting a case about safe sex in relation to larger issues of sexual rights, pointing out that "if you are having sex and you are not spreading the virus it doesn't matter if you have sex with one person or ten thousand". If listened to, this statement simply blasts Chapman's position into smithereens. So it is not listened to, the voice-over merely commenting, "so you don't think homosexuals need to alter the practice of having a lot of partners to prevent the virus spreading?", unable to realise that there is not a uniform category of "homosexuals" with "the practice of having a lot of partners", or that the number of one's sexual partners is not intrinsically a moral question at all, and would only become so in relation to questions of consent and honesty. Nor, of course, has she registered the fact that monogamy is no more of an immediate protection from Aids than is prayer, or fasting. Aids is not contracted by promiscuity, but by blood, which is common even to moral paragons such as Ms Chapman. She, however, sails on regardless of such trivial niceties, arguing that "not all gays agree with this defence of homosexual behaviour", a comment all the more revealing and hypocritical since nobody besides herself had so much as intimated that "homosexual behaviour" requires any "defence". One man with Aids was trotted on to say that "this sort of message only encourages gays to take risks", which is highly disputable, but the main witness for the prosecution was ready in the wings to put a much stronger case – one Graham Hancock, described only as the author of *Aids: The Deadly Epidemic*, which is not exactly a title to inspire instant respect and confidence.

Hancock's premise is simple: "To advocate promiscuity, to advocate furtherance of the main way in which this virus is transmitted, is to advocate genocide". After all, there's nothing quite like a bit of good old fashioned British understatement, and another gay person with Aids is instantly conjured up to repeat the message. The "respectable" middle-aged woman then reappears to venture the dangerous opinion that she doesn't accept that she ever was promiscuous, since one always sees oneself as the norm of sexual behaviour. But such cautious sense is quickly dispatched by Mr Hancock's words that "the whole of society is now a risk group. The more sexual partners you have, the more likely you are to come into contact with the disease". Ms Chapman then reappears to cross-examine the government's chief medical officer, Dr Donald Acheson, accusing him of having failed to inform the nation about the need for absolute monogamy, a charge of which he is, of course, found guilty and disposed of, to be replaced by the reliable Hancock, insisting incorrectly yet again that "this is a sexually transmitted disease", as if this ended debate. Then, against a highly selective roll-call of legislation since the 1960s, Chapman asks "If the best protection against this disease is monogamy" (which it is *not*) "why are we so reluctant to say it? Is the fear of being called a moralist worse than the fear of Aids itself?" Evidently not for Ms Chapman, who now proceeds with a sinister re-reading of modern history, according to which,

> "a progressive consensus, supported by twenty years of legislation, says moral behaviour is our own private business. Anyone who disagrees is simply anti-permissive. But with Aids around, can we afford the luxury of these views?"

This is frankly terrifying nonsense. To begin with, it offers a spectacularly bizarre reading of recent history, as if "privacy" has been zealously protected from institutional interference of any kind since the 1960s, and simply lines us up to a crude "anti-permissive" position which refuses any debate. Another doctor, and then another gay person with Aids are spliced in to support the case, the latter criticising "the old Seventies attitudes of sleeping around and experimentation, and it's alright... without bringing in Victorian morality, to perhaps say that it's OK to be monogamous". The point here is simply that it's never *not* been OK to be monogamous. As I have argued, "promiscuity" and "monogamy" are not helpful terms with which to think complex moral issues about sexual diversity, least of all at a time when programmes like this are busily trying to persuade us that sex, and gay sex in particular, is not only dirty, but deadly. Now, more than ever, gay men need to affirm their collective sexual identity, safely, and without shame or the type of guilt which Chapman and her ilk so shamelessly set out to exploit – choosing sick, frightened, and possibly dying men to parrot her single and catastrophically misguided *idée fixe*.

The programme ends with Ms Chapman, discovered seated in a laboratory of some kind, once more smiling like a villain, to announce that

> "Aids... says we can no longer enjoy sexual freedom without seriously damaging our health, and the lives of others. Unfortunately it's very unlikely that you'll hear that said, so we've made our own television advert to sell the message".

The advert was a nightmare. "Spooky" music preludes five figures, lit from behind, in a dark blank studio space. "Which one of these people can give you Aids if you sleep with them?" asks a husky mid-Atlantic male voice, earnestly, as the camera tracks across a mildly punkish boy of about twenty, a female "secretary" type, a woman "of a certain age", a young man in a plaid shirt, and a slightly older man wearing a suit. Their faces are then scrambled by a computer and recombined and revolved through 365° as if on an identity parade which, of course, they are. "You can't tell? No, you can't tell from looking. Aids doesn't choose other people. Aids can choose you". We then cut to a stark title which reads AIDS KILLS in large white letters, above MAKE IT MONOGAMY in red. Aids, however, doesn't "choose" anyone, nor does it "say" anything. It is simply there for Ms Chapman to exploit, though she seems to have forgotten that British television won't broadcast any adverts which are construed as sexually direct.

A month before this programme was shown, Mrs Mary Whitehouse, President of the National Viewers' and Listeners' Association, expressed "anxiety" about the mere possibility of a magazine format programme for lesbians and gay men, currently being mooted by Channel Four.

> "It is essential," [she said] "for everybody's sake, that before these programmes are shown they are most closely scrutin-ised for any verbal or visual element which could make gay appear normal or in any way to be recommended ... everything possible must be done to protect the public from this new and terrible threat".[14]

The "everybody" in this formulation obviously excludes lesbians and gay men. As Peter Tatchell has noted:

> "When Aids was only killing homosexuals she never showed the slightest interest or concern. From someone who proclaims that homosexuality 'is not normal or in any way to be recommended' perhaps such ignorance and neglect is only to be expected".[15]

Much the same could be said of Christine Chapman, and the BBC's *Horizon* team, and a host of other television journalists and commentators who cannot see beyond the national family unit, which constitutes the miserably impoverished core of television's understanding of its actual audience. In the face of ever increasingly direct state interference in the workings of British and American television, lesbians and gay men need more than ever to insist, in the words of George Eliot, that "our passions do not live apart in locked chambers". We must listen and attend very closely to what television has to say about Aids with all its many voices. For in the coming years it will be increasingly important that we are able calmly and confidently to answer back and lobby an institution which claims to know us in advance, and has an almost limitless capacity to frame and edit us in such a way that we are heard to speak its truths, and its values, as if they were our own. We need to be able to reply with Jean Genet, who, when asked by an imbecile from the BBC if he had a first lover at Reform School, paused, and then said: "No. Two hundred."[16]

Chapter Seven

Safer representations

Personal reactions to having Aids are unpredictable. An Aids diagnosis may lead to an immediate sense of relief that things are out in the open, named and therefore resistable, or to an equally immediate sense of stark, paralysing terror. From somewhere between the two a close friend wrote to me:

> "Overall, I have good days and bad days, mentally... it's like a nightmare, I'm mostly anguished by a sense of complete unbelievability. I keep wanting to wake up and it's June again and none of this has happened – because 'of course' only nightmares are like this."

Edmund White has described how, after taking the HIV antibody test with his boy friend, he was told he was "positive" and his boy friend "negative":

> "We then went off for a romantic trip to Vienna which had already been planned. I just wept the whole time. I didn't want him to go through it all, felt I was being irrational, would get up, go to the bathroom, cry and then come back. Finally he realised what was happening and was sweet and reassuring... Every gay couple I know is going through something like this. I know we're not alone in this kind of suffering."[1]

White, however, is unusual in so far as he has chosen to go "public", unlike any other gay celebrity whose reputation extends beyond the territory of gay culture.

This is not to imply that anyone should necessarily "come out" as antibody-positive. It is obviously a complex and extremely difficult personal decision, and an attack on the late Michel Foucault in the *New York Native* for not having "come out" with Aids before he died was as insensitive to the situation of all other people with Aids as it was morally indefensible in relation to Foucault. The vast majority of gay people with Aids have no hope, however, of penetrating the thick carapace established throughout the mass media in the form of the agenda set for what people with Aids are like – who they are, where they come from, how they live, and what they think and feel. The fetishising of monogamy as the "answer" to Aids ensures the representational obliteration of lives which do not accept the terms of the host cultures which silence them. In this respect a discourse of punitive fidelity has been imposed in the name of monogamy on those whose sexuality eludes the restrictive model of marriage as a sacrament, binding on individuals regardless of all ethical, psychic, social or sexual factors.

This discourse of punitive fidelity constructs three pictures of people with Aids. On the one hand we hear repeatedly of "Aids victims" who have been abandoned by their families, but more especially by gay friends and lovers. Whilst it would be pointless to pretend that this has never happened, it nonetheless remains intensely significant that one of the only ways in which we are invited to think of the situation of gay people with Aids is as victims of one another, or of their own communities. Thus attention is deflected away from the real rejection on the part of governments, hospitals, welfare organisations, as well as the mass media. Secondly, we are presented with the figure of the "irresponsible" gay man, stalking out into the night to put other men at risk. These are the gay men who allegedly "refuse" the warnings so kindly offered by the press and on television, and who are unwilling to "change their ways". Lastly, we are offered the whispered voices of broken men, disclosed in lonely bedsits and hospital isolation wards, hoarsely and desperately repeating the "need" for monogamy, in tones of deep regret and not infrequently of self-recrimination and blame. These constitute the saddest spectacle, men who have been recruited to accept the status of the "guilty victim". Their exploitation is all the more unpleasant since they are invariably used in place of the majority of unapologetic and affirmatively identified people with Aids who so courageously reject the imagery of hopelessness.

These are the figures who mediate Aids to the rest of the population, the motifs which represent the syndrome and supposedly reflect its "truth" in the public places of the mass communications industry. However, as Stuart Hall argues,

> "representation is a very different notion from that of reflection. It implies the active work of selecting and presenting, of structuring and shaping: not merely the transmitting of already-existing meaning, but the more active labour of *making things mean*".[2]

It is the hard, sustained, and largely unconscious work of representation which produces the effect of a society which is only fully intelligible from within the heterosexual family unit. The mere existence of positively identified and sexually affirmative lesbians and gay men constantly threatens to reveal the ponderous and laborious machinery of cultural heterosexualisation right across the media. Which is why our every appearance is so carefully policed in a system of representational checks and balances to establish our essential "perversity". Journalists and television reporters inevitably appear to lesbians and gay men as Wizards of Oz, the wheels and levers of their power baldly exposed in the space between our lived experience, and the representations made of us in the media. We cannot say that such representations "influence" other people, unless we assume that human subjectivity is formed prior to and independent of the workings of words and images. On the contrary, the power of the media lies in its capacity to manufacture subjectivity itself.

The flash-point of conflict between desire, and the various institutions which regulate the look of the social world, is the human body. We can see this conflict very sharply in the chimera of pornography. For anti-porn campaigners,

> "there is a social and psychic link between pornography and rape. In terms of patriarchal morality, both are expressions of male lust, which is presumed to be innately vicious, and offensive to the putative sexual innocence of the 'good' woman".[3]

In order to persuade us that explicit sexual imagery leads to sexual violence in a simple, one-to-one manner, the anti-porn lobby requires the crudest and most reductive reflection theory of how words and images work. Thus porn is held to "reflect" male sexuality, and to "cause" sexual aggression. Since it only takes a moment's thought to realise that if male sexuality were intrinsically violent it wouldn't need the trigger of pornography, we may safely deduce that these arguments are not available to rational solution. Those who invariably refuse to acknowledge the constant negotiation of meanings on television or in newspapers by readers and viewers are always those who wish to exercise absolute control over what the rest of us may read or watch.

In this context the exuberant confidence of lesbian and gay male sexuality will inevitably seem at odds with the familial moralism of the mass media. Our frankness and articulacy and sheer gaiety disturbs the poky, repressive little world-of-the-family, and threatens to expose the brutal forces which hold it together across the entire field of "public" representations. These forces may be backed by legislation, but they do not necessarily originate from the state. They all subscribe, however, to a system of inherited historical explanations and beliefs about "human nature". This idea of nature is organised at its most fundamental in relation to the body, and to the distinction between male and female bodies, and adult and childish bodies, and what is held to be appropriate to each. The entire structure of "official" representations in the West proceeds from this set of distinctions, which are the prerequisite for the workings of all other power relations. It is therefore important that individuals should recognise themselves in these terms and their derived images, since they constitute the very ground on which the family has emerged, as Michel Foucault argues, "as an element internal to population, and as a fundamental instrument of its government".[4]

The relations of male to female, and adult to child, are assumed to be symmetrical and reciprocal, in such a way that homosexuality appears as a failure rather than a variant of sexual reciprocity, an asymmetry which disrupts what are held to be immutable categories. These are most intimately inscribed in anxieties about physical contact, and the rules which derive from them about exactly which parts of different people's bodies may never touch. Thus men can shake hands, or slap one another on the back. They can hug on football pitches, and shower together after the game. In France they may even kiss. But they are not allowed to touch one another's penises under any circumstances, nor must they admit to any sensual or erotic pleasure from the touch or sight of one another's bodies. Above all they must not fuck or suck together. These rules about what is "appropriate" also apply to individual parts of the body, and are enforced from earliest childhood, lining up the body towards the adult world of labour, and the opposite sex. So, whilst we eat and talk and kiss with our mouths, our genitals are subject to much more rigorously functionalist regulation. That the male rectum is the most thoroughly policed part of the male anatomy suggests that a particular effort is needed to redirect the libido away from deeply repressed memories of anal erotic pleasure in infancy, at a time when our primary awareness of our bodies is erotogenic. Aids offers a new sign for the symbolic machinery of repression, making the rectum a grave. At this point the categories of health and sickness, by which we also know our bodies, meet with those of sex, and the image of homosexuality is re-inscribed with connotations of contagion and disease, a subject for medical attention and medical authority. Thus promiscuity has become at last a primarily medical term, just as morality has been effectively medicalised.

This is why the representation of Aids seems so starkly anachronistic: gay sex, read as "promiscuous", is being medically redefined as unsafe. Aids takes us back to the pre-modern world, with disease restored to its ancient theological status as punishment. Therefore it is most important to question the systematic mis-classification of Aids as a Sexually Transmitted Disease (henceforth

STD). For although the HIV virus is primarily acquired through sex, this does not mean that it is primarily an STD. As Kaye Wellings of the Family Planning Association observes:

> "To include in the category those diseases which 'can be transmitted' makes the category so large as to be meaningless. If all conditions that could be transmitted sexually were included, then the common cold might well find itself being dealt with in STD clinics".[5]

The entire representation of Aids hangs upon the ways in which, as she points out, "medicine has been used to normalise sexual conduct".[6] This is the perspective from which we read of the "Aids virus", a phrase which falsely telescopes and concentrates the entire context of the disease into a narrow alignment with specific sexual acts. Hence the plethora of medical explanations which proceeded from the assumption that there must be something about gay sex as such which rendered so many gay men vulnerable to infection. These "explanations" included the supposedly "immuno-suppressive nature" of sperm, and the still more obviously homophobic notion that the mere possibility of blood to sperm contact might be responsible. Needless to say, such explanations would find it difficult to account for the survival of a high proportion of people of both sexes enjoying anal sex over the course of human history.

The fact that an incurable virus has invaded our communities cannot be blamed on gay sex as such, though the situation is exacerbated by the fact that we both fuck and get fucked, thus running a high risk of both absorbing infected sperm, and passing it on. Edmund White has used this same observation to argue against explanations of Aids which attribute it to gay "promiscuity". But I do not think this is particularly helpful, since it is obvious that gay culture has enabled us to enjoy sex, and not feel guilty about it, and not always to equate love with lifelong sexual fidelity to one person. This has been the strength of our culture, not its weakness. In any case it remains far from clear that gay men talking about sex, and moralists talking about sex, are actually referring to the same thing. For the moralist sex is a thing you do, an act, with a limited duration and a clear performance principle. For most gay men, however, sex involves a far broader degree of general eroticised physical contact, in which fucking and sucking are episodes of intimacy among others. As Robert Glück has written of pre-Aids bath-house sex in San Francisco: "We watch the pleasure rather than the men, feeling the potential interchangeability".[7] Gay sex is about maximising the mutual erotic possibilities of the body, and that is why it is taboo. It comes too close to the infant's experience of polymorphous perversity – deriving potential sexual pleasure from every part of itself and its surroundings – which is so violently repressed in the formation of orthodox adult sexualities.

In this manner powerful social *and* psychic factors combine to frame Aids as a product of sexual "excess", in terms of quantity and quality. Firm statistics showing the distribution of the virus amongst gay men are impossible to come by, since those coming forward for antibody testing are likely to have done so from a perception of risk which already distinguishes them from most men on the gay scene in Britain. For reasons which I have already touched on, there is little or no equivalent in the UK to the American range of gay identities, since homosexuality here is always in competition with other identities, of class, race and regionalism, all competing for ascendancy. Whilst this ensures that homosexuality is more broadly integrated into other areas of social consciousness, by the same token it also means that gay men have a much weaker sense of collective interest than in the United States. The situation of British gay men is far more atomised than that of our American contemporaries, and we are far more closely subject to immediate and direct regulation, ranging from licensing laws, legal prohibitions against bath-houses, and the enforced absence of anything remotely resembling the sex-affirmative cultural institutions which flourish in America. The disco revolution of the early 1970s has now atrophied into a deafening inferno of hi-energy muzak. The majority of gay pubs are still owned by breweries who have no interest in their clientele beyond issues of profitability. Pubs and clubs alike have signally failed to take any initiatives on behalf of the very people who have no choice but to use their services, given the close invigilation of alcohol licences by the police, which effectively forbids the possibility of an autonomous large-scale gay social scene. There are no national publications remotely comparable to the *Advocate* or the *New York Native* in America, or *Gai Pied* in France, or *The Body Politic* in Canada. British gay men are extraordinarily cut off from other national gay cultures, and in the absence of a local gay press of any seriousness, have little access to information about Aids beyond what is available in the national dailies, and on television. This is the baleful situation in which any realistic discussion of safe sex must be set.

By definition, epidemiology is about statistics. The statistical likelihood of contracting the HIV virus from a new sexual partner in New York is now put at fifty-fifty, and up to five per cent for women. Counselling monogamy as an end in itself in such a context is simply putting the cart before the horse, since monogamous sex is no safer than any other kind, especially if you're gay and potentially at risk of contracting the virus from anyone who's had sex in the last seven years. In a purely statistical sense it could be argued that immediate and total punitive fidelity would lead to something less than an exact doubling of HIV infection, since many people with the virus would presumably end up with partners in the same situation. Then, according to this logic, the situation would be contained. But sex is not about statistics, and punitive fidelity would inevitably produce sexual counteraction, even if it could in any way be effectively policed. Besides, sexuality is intrinsically caught up in unconscious circuits of abandon and denial, desire and resistance. Changes in sexual behaviour cannot be forced, they can only be achieved through consent, consent which incorporates change into the very structure of sexual fantasy. Hence the urgent, the desperate need to eroticise information about safe sex, if tens of thousands of more lives are not to be cruelly sacrificed on the twin altars of prudery and homophobia.

At the best of times, public information about sex is pitifully inadequate. Persistent government interference in education has denied generations of children access to adequate information about the world in which they grow up. In the name of "protection", children are forcibly maintained in a state of ignorance, fear, and vulgar prejudice about their own and other people's sexuality. A gay teenager in a London school has told me of the scale of private persecution which is his everyday life as an openly gay pupil. He is shunned, spat upon and reviled as an "Aids carrier". His situation is perhaps analogous to that of a German boy in an English school in the early days of the Second World War. He is fortunate, in so far as he is part of a supportive group of gay teenagers. But thousands like him find themselves isolated and vulnerable to the heatwave of hatred generated against gay men in recent years by the British press. Whilst it is easy for liberals to laugh at the rantings of the *Sun*, and even documentaries on the BBC, it behoves us to take their prejudice very seriously indeed, since they help determine the climate in which decisions about matters of life and death must be made. To many of us the quaint moralism of government ministers and newspaper owners and the directors of British radio and television may indeed seem laughable. Yet power lies with these people. Priorities are now being set at the Medical Research Council, which has already suffered from serious government cuts in funding, about the future management of this epidemic. Aids could easily be made a notifiable disease in Britain. But hospitals are already chronically understaffed and overworked. Aids thus raises the whole question of a government's responsibilities to provide adequate health care for a nation's citizens. It casts a strong light on the consequences of cuts in National Health Service expenditure under the Thatcher regime, just as it focuses attention on the iniquity of private medicine in the United States.

The British government has spent more than two million pounds on a public information campaign about Aids which does not even begin to scratch the surface of the problem. Until recently it gave a mere one hundred thousand pounds per annum to The Terrence Higgins Trust, the only British Aids charity large enough even to contemplate the task of reaching perhaps two million men in the UK with information that can save their lives. The annual running costs of the Trust are more than one quarter of a million pounds, from which it also finances a part-time telephone service, counselling, administrative work, hospital "buddy" services – all the most difficult human needs which this epidemic has brought into being. There is a fight against Aids going on in the research laboratories of France, Britain and America, a fight which is stimulated by the prospect of enormous financial profits, and professional awards. There is also another fight taking place, as volunteers hand out free condoms at gay discos, talk to people in pubs, try to spread the word that people can protect themselves and one another. But with "only" 500 deaths in what is a highly fragmented and disparate constituency, direct experience of Aids is still very rare. In Bristol and Norwich, Aids is widely associated with London, just as in London it is associated with New York. In a world, as Auden described it, where "few people accept each other and most will never do anything properly",[8] rumour is unlikely to galvanise people into casually changing the sexual pleasures of a lifetime overnight. And who would listen to "advice" from a government and a political system that has the greatest difficulty in even acknowledging the existence of homosexuality, except as a target for increasingly punitive legislation.

Whilst STD clinics give away free condoms, other doctors can ask publicly in print if we can "allow thousands of Aids victims to assume the major proportion of hospital beds for what is primarily a self-inflicted disease",[9] and remind a nurse looking after a man weighing only four stone and dying in agony that "what you forget is that he is the architect of his own misfortune".[10] Professor Anthony Pinching and others have pointed out the straightforward ineffectiveness of moralising at people: "Every person with Aids or HIV (HTLV3) infection is a human tragedy. Every case of HIV transmission prevented is a triumph". Criticising Mr John McKay, the Scottish Minister of Health, Professor Pinching concludes

> "I cannot understand a moral stance that is not only unmoved by disease and death, but actually allows one to

stand by, arrogantly inactive in the face of expert advice, when one has the power to prevent them".[11]

He favours the distribution of condoms, and needles and syringes for IV drug-users. Yet he is arguing against the modern equivalents of the National Council for combating Venereal Disease, which refused to offer advice on contraceptives in the early decades of this century on the grounds that this would provide some kind of incentive to "immoral" behaviour. As long ago as August, 1983, the *Medical News* reported under the heading "Homosexuals advised to use condoms to prevent AIDS" that

> "A condom may not appear to be the essential item of equipment for a practising homosexual. But many homosexuals may have to consider their routine use, according to a theory proposed by Anne McLaren of the Medical Research Council Mammalian Development Unit in London."

Unlike many other AIDS stories in the medical press, newspapers did not pick that one up. Nor, it seems, did anyone else at the time. And even now, as I have shown, the prospect of total celibacy is held up to save lives, rather than a condom.

It seems to me that several things need to be done if people are to take to safe sex without resistance. Firstly, talk of "risk groups", and the banding together of degrees of risk from different sexual practices within such groups, needs to be dropped, since it inevitably implies that most people, gay or straight, are not at risk. They are. Secondly, we need to think about Smart Sex as much as Safer Sex, in the words of Dr Barbara Stanett at a rally protesting against the reporting policy of the *New York Post* in the winter of 1985. We will not improve matters by treating people like children, and employing similar strategies to those we rightly deplore in the straight press. The recognition of the need for collective care and responsibility will not emerge from didactic flourishes. How can we expect other people to take themselves and one another seriously, if we do not address them seriously in the first place? Thirdly, we need to avoid mythifying Aids. The situation of the person with Aids is not poignant, not at all like a poem by Cavafy, or a Donizetti opera, or a Gershwin song. Heroising those who have lived longest with the syndrome only reinforces an attitude towards statistics and average life expectancies which no individual should be expected to identify their case with. This can only too easily lead to a subtle type of blaming those who are not so fortunate in their experience of the syndrome. It is equally important that "alternative" medical therapy does not simply trade in the experience of orthodox medicine for a "patient-centred" approach which still manages to blame people with Aids in the context of their whole lifestyle. The greatest achievement of all the various organisations supporting and caring for people with Aids has been the assertion of affirmative attitudes towards life and health. As John Keats wrote to his sister Fanny in 1820:

> "I am sorry to hear you have been so ill and in such low spirits. Now you are better, keep so. Do not suffer your mind to dwell on unpleasant reflections ... There are enough real distresses and evils in wait for every one to try the most vigorous health ... Do not diet your mind with grief, it destroys the constitution; but let your chief care be of your health, and with that you will meet your share of pleasure in the world – do not doubt it".[12]

Fourthly, we need to develop a culture which will support the transition to safer sex by establishing the model of an erotics of protection, succour and support within the framework of our pre-Aids sex lives. Books like John Preston's *Hot Living* offer a start for thinking about how we can make the most of where people are actually coming from, sexually, rather than disregarding it altogether.[13] We must not collude with the anti-sex lobby all around us, for it is precisely their equation of sex with Aids which stands to construct a new contagion theory of homosexuality which is every bit as tenacious as that which has taken us the better part of a century to successfully dismantle. Hence the inappropriateness of a recent article aimed at young gays which ended with a pious wish that "hopefully our imaginary gay teenager will never miss what he's never had, and a new generation of gay men will learn to live without fucking".[14] Whilst newspaper owners and the authorities regulating television refuse to allow the ordinary advertising of condoms, let alone erotic adverts for safer gay sex, it is up to gay men to press for changes in the laws regulating public representations of gay sexuality. But there would be little point in exchanging the situation in which gay sex can only be spoken as transgression, for another situation in which gay sex is identified only as a possible source of infection. If sex were not pleasurable people would not be at risk, and we cannot help people consider risks if we deny all pleasure in sex. This is why we need to return, in conclusion, to the question of fantasy.

Fantasy "is not the object of desire, but its setting".[15] It is through the mobilisation of fantasy that we can protect ourselves from the risk of infection as well as against the threatening re-homosexualisation of our entire culture – a culture which in Britain is particularly fragile. As one Australian Aids counsellor has argued:

"We have to be very careful not to create the impression in the minds of gay men that gay sex is, in itself, dangerous, unhealthy, unsafe, or anything else negative. That's the attitude that has produced some of the gibbering wrecks that we see in this office. If we do this, if we make people *afraid* to be gay, we will not only poison the roots of our existence as a community, we will also actually harm the people we are trying to help, by creating quite unnecessary stress and anxiety, on top of the unavoidable stress already caused by the epidemic ... We should make it clear that the purpose of our information effort is to make good sex better, by making it safer, rather than to make safe sex seem boring, complicated, or something only prudes or wimps are interested in".[16]

To expect anyone, or any group of people, completely to renounce desire is simply to invite feelings of guilt and low self-esteem, and the repressed is only too likely to return in the form of extremely unsafe sex indeed.

What we need to establish is a sex education campaign aimed at gay men in the form of "compromise-formations", which would permit what is understood as the loss of certain sexual pleasures to be sublimated in relation to gains at the level of fantasy. By definition, satisfactions which are withdrawn only stimulate desire. This is why we so urgently need to enlarge and expand our sense of the sexual, in order to incorporate condoms as new stage props into the theatre of our desiring fantasies. We can explore precisely those aspects of our sexuality which are in a sense "dangerous", but which do not expose us to any risk of infection – voyeurism for example, exhibitionism, and all the ways in which we escape that central fear of sexual difference which so cripples much of heterosexual culture, as epitomised in its pornographic imaginings. We need to organise huge regular Safe Sex parties in our clubs and gay centres, as have been held in many Dutch cities, with workshops and expert counselling available.[17] We need to produce hot, sexy visual materials to take home, telephone sex-talk facilities, and safe sex porno cinemas. All discotheques, youth clubs and other centres of youth culture should be obliged to provide Safer Sex information for all their clients. We need a massive television campaign about the use of condoms targeted at all the constituencies of desire which actually make up the population. We need a poster campaign across the length and breadth of the British Isles reminding people to use condoms, on a par with long-standing Scandinavian policy and practice. We need free disposable needles distributed to IV drug-users. We need – as an

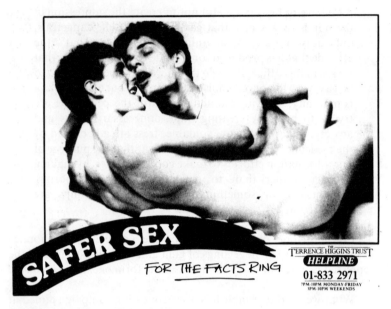

The Terrence Higgins Trust, leaflet

absolute priority – to have a national HIV antibody testing service which is totally anonymous and confidential, and an extensive national counselling service which would be adequate to the enormous task of supporting those found to be infected.

Above all, we need adequate financing. The Terrence Higgins Trust is to date the only organisation actively communicating Safer Sex advice and information to women and IV drug-users, as well as gay men, yet its annual budget is not fixed well in advance. It is not reasonable or practical to expect voluntary organisations to carry the entire load of public information campaigning on top of the vital and difficult one-to-one role of counselling the thousands of individuals who have either tested positive or who have Aids. In other words, we need to create a whole new post-Aids culture, geared to the specific needs of the times, a culture of collective sexual affirmation which respects diversity and is dedicated to developing a sense of mutual responsibility which alone will save lives. To this end we need to abandon the insane notion that Aids is only a threat to "risk" communities, without neglecting the very specific rights and needs of gay men, who have been most devastated by this catastrophe. Governments must heed the experience of those who have social as well as medical expertise. The executive director of New York's Gay

Men's Health Crisis has stated bluntly that "health education is the only tool that can stem this epidemic".[18] Ann Guidici Fettner, who is the finest American medical correspondent writing on Aids, has recently observed that "Aids education should have started the moment it was realised that this disease is sexually transmitted".[19] The mass media's wilful construction of Aids as a "Gay Plague" has perfectly complemented government inaction and already guaranteed the death of thousands of people in Britain by the end of the decade. In these circumstances we should recall Thucydides' bracingly laconic observation on the great plague of Athens, written more than two thousand years ago: "As for the gods, it seemed to be the same thing whether one worshipped them or not, when one saw the good and the bad dying indiscriminately".[20] Until gay men are provided with the same health facilities as other citizens in this present emergency, it will be difficult not to conclude that we are regarded in our entirety as a disposable population.

Epilogue

Shortly after the main text of this book had gone to press, the British government announced its commitment to a "forceful" new propaganda campaign "to alert the public to the risks of Aids".[1] Advertisements spelled out the word "AIDS" in seasonal gift wrapping paper, together with the accompanying question: "How many people will get it for Christmas?". Another advert conveys the message that "Your next sexual partner could be that very special person" – framed inside a heart, like a Valentine – with a supplement beneath which tersely adds, "The one that gives you Aids". The official line is clearly anti-sex, and draws on an assumed rhetoric from previous Aids commentary concerning "promiscuity" as the supposed "cause" of Aids. A series of huge hoardings has also appeared throughout Britain, with their messages seemingly carved into granite-like tomb-stones. Thus we read the solemn injunction, "AIDS: DON'T DIE OF IGNORANCE", with the secondary information that "Anyone can get it, gay or straight, male or female. Already 30,000 people are infected. At the moment the infection is *mainly confined to relatively small groups of people* in this country. But it is spreading."

According to the most recently published statistics, there have been 731 cases of Aids in Britain so far, of whom 377 have already died. Of the total figure, twenty-five are heterosexual, of whom five contracted the virus via heterosexual sex.[2] Something very strange indeed is going on behind the government campaign. At first sight it seems actually to acknowledge the diversity of sexuality in the modern world. Yet this is clearly not the case, since we are obviously intended to dismiss all thought of the vast majority of people with Aids as members of "relatively small groups". At the same time the poster projects a mischievous implication of responsibility onto people who already have Aids, as if they'd set out to contract the HIV virus by ignoring information which, as I have shown, has never been widely available. In other words it has taken only five cases of Aids caused by heterosexual sex to throw the government into a frenzy of public activity. Apart from lesbians and gay men, which other social group with over 700 dead and dying, could have been so totally and cynically erased from all public consideration?

Another poster proclaims, "AIDS IS NOT PREJUDICED: IT CAN KILL ANYONE", with the sub-heading: "It's true more men than women have Aids, but this does not mean it is a homosexual disease. It isn't". Here we find the astonishing implication that there is indeed such a thing as a virus which selects its victims according to their sexuality, or at least that some diseases are intrinsic to gay men, even if Aids is *not* one of them. Since the obvious opportunity to point out that there is simply no such thing as a virus which is gender-specific, and only affects men *or* women has not been taken up, it is only possible to conclude that what the poster actually says is that it doesn't matter if you *are* prejudiced – just as long as you don't make the mistake of thinking that Aids is "only" killing off the queers!

Yet another poster screams out, "THE LONGER YOU BELIEVE AIDS ONLY AFFECTS OTHERS, THE FASTER IT'LL SPREAD". Here, as usual, Aids is collapsed into the HIV virus, with the totally incorrect implication that Aids itself is actively infectious. This inability to distinguish clearly between Aids and the HIV virus demonstrates the immediate shortcomings of an approach to health education which also refuses to recognise and respond to the actual diversity of the total population, according to the distinctions of class, age, race, gender, religion or sexual orientation. The worst poster of all coyly offers the question, "AIDS: HOW MUCH BIGGER DOES IT HAVE TO GET BEFORE YOU TAKE NOTICE?". The question however which we should *all* be asking some six years into this epidemic is how large did *it* have to get before *they* took any notice? The folly and tragedy of this entire campaign lies in its rejection of all but the most general and over-abstracted approaches to health education, whilst doing nothing whatsoever to counter the torrents of media misinformation which have preceded it by many years.

The leaflet which has gone out to every household in Britain shares the same obituary graphics as the poster campaign, and whilst it contains a great deal of straightforward factual information which challenges the picture of Aids as a contagious condition, it nonetheless proceeds from an initial statement that Aids is "not just a homosexual disease". This is a shocking and disgraceful statement in a supposedly democratic society where governments are supposed to protect the rights of all subjects. If anyone still doubts that gay men are officially regarded, in our entirety, as a disposable constituency, they need read no further. Millions of pounds have been spent on a crude loud-hailing exercise which directs itself to nobody in particular, and least of all to those most urgently in need of positive, supportive health education. This is why the didactic call not "to die of ignorance" is so insufferable, coming from a government which has efficiently kept gay men in ignorance about Aids throughout the 1980s and which regards us only as a target for ever more punitive legislation, prosecution, and surveillance.

In the meantime two men with Aids have already been burned out of their own homes in one borough of London alone[3] and the new mood of national Aids awareness remains propped up by the ignorance and prejudice of the newspaper industry and many politicians. Mortal fears have been whipped up, as if sexuality and sexual desire were entirely within the control of rational consciousness, with the first groups affected by the virus still being widely held as its direct cause. Nothing whatsoever has been done at any official level in either Britain or the United States to challenge the endlessly repeated media association between homosexuality *per se* and Aids. Nor is anything of the kind likely to be forthcoming in the forseeable future from the recently established Health Education Authority in Britain, which has been set up to manage the treatment of people with Aids, as well as the next stages of the official national campaign. Indeed, the first public statement, on a radio chat show, by its Director, Ann Burdus, hardly augurs well for the future, since she arrogantly dismissed anyone involved with questions of gay rights as "lunatics". Ms Burdus compensates for her total former innocence of any involvement with issues of health education by having been a previous winner of the Veuve Cliquot Businesswoman of The Year award, and an ex. chairman (*sic.*) and Chief Executive of McCann Erickson, one of Britain's largest advertising agencies.

In the meantime the Government campaign has stimulated a number of unintended but inevitable consequences, and its ambiguities and defects are clearly revealed from the contradictory ways in which the British newspaper industry and network television have responded to it. Both have used it as a licence of kinds, but to widely differing objectives. One of the most striking consequences of the overall campaign lies precisely in the manner in which it has sent the press and television hurtling off in radically different directions. This is not to assume that either press or television coverage are themselves entirely coherent. Nonetheless it is apparent that two new agendas for thinking about Aids are currently emerging, and that 1987 marks the first real shift in Aids commentary since the epidemic first hit the international headlines in 1983. Both, however, are mutations of the earlier stages of Aids commentary which I have described and analysed.

The British Press is currently enthusiastically following up the "lead" of the American Murdoch-owned newspapers, which have long been calling for mass testing and the quarantine of people with Aids, with an entirely predictable knock-on effect amongst their

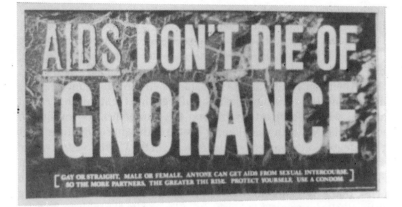

rivals. It should be noted from the outset that the British press still depends *in its entirety* on three fundamentally misleading notions in its coverage of Aids. First, the idea of an "Aids-virus", which condenses the distinct and crucial distinction between HIV infection and Aids. Second, the notion of an "Aids-carrier", which follows on from the idea of an "Aids-virus", whilst making it impossible to distinguish between people with HIV infection, and people with Aids. At the same time it falsely imputes to both groups the completely inaccurate connotations of contagious illness, in an ancient but still highly potent rhetoric of plague-carriers, with strong implications of direct risk and threat to the rest of the population. Third, the Press talks of the "Aids test", whilst never for one moment stopping to establish either the nature, or purposes, of the HIV antibody test. The absolutely fundamental point to bear in mind through all of this is that there is *no such thing* as "the Aids virus", or an "Aids carrier", or "the Aids test". That these three points are not basic common knowledge, is the measure of the *total* and *absolute* irresponsibility of the British media, in all its hydra forms and variants. Having temporarily run out of steam in their tiring competition to invent ever more lurid and sensationalist stories concerning Aids, the newspaper industry is now busily establishing a new agenda which seeks to mobilise public opinion behind calls for medically indefensible measures and above all, I suspect, for the recriminalisation of homosexuality. An early indication of this shift appeared in Charles Maclean's report for the *Evening Standard* on 2 February, where he stated that, "incredibly, the New York Board of Health has never officially designated Aids as a communicable disease". Whilst this is *literally* true, it is not in the least incredible, but remains on the contrary a matter for fervent relief – and a sign that American health authorities, like their British counterparts – understand the social implications of legal interventions in medical affairs, which seem utterly beyond the comprehension of British journalists. Maclean calculatedly obscures the entire significance of the category of "communicable" disease in the United States, where all cases of Aids are reported to the Center for Disease Control in Atlanta, Georgia. They are not, however, "communicable" in the sense that PWAs are not then subject to American laws concerning officially "communicable" diseases, allowing local health authorities to apply restrictions ranging from house arrrest to enforced confinement in isolation hospitals. Only certain contagious diseases have been designated as officially "communicable" in the past – and neither HIV nor Aids are, of course, contagious. Maclean's purpose is evidently mischievous and sinister in the extreme, and represents a new press campaign to pressurise the British government into making Aids an officially notifiable disease, with identical consequences over here as for those with communicable illnesses in the USA. This campaign is clearly punitive in its aspect to PWAs, and aims to exploit what journalists and editors alike clearly perceive as widespread hatred and fear of gay men, who make up the majority of Aids cases in the USA as in Britain. Hence the strategic use of polls and phone-ins, which permit newspapers to project their own policies in such a way that they seem to derive directly from readers – understood as the "great British public", supposedly one hundred per cent heterosexual.

Thus in a more recent readers' survey for the *Sun*, reporter Peter Cliff asked whether "You The Jury" (note the implication of *judgement*) thinks that everyone going into hospital should be tested for HIV, alongside an editorial concluding that "this is a sensible idea. But it would not be at all sensible to keep the results secret" on the grounds that a positive test result makes a person instantly a "menace". Cliff, whom connoisseurs of Aids journalism may recall as the author of last year's *Sun* scorcher, "My Misery Posing As An AIDS Victim" (the *Sun*, 23 January, 1986), received his phone-in poll results next day, with 2,866 readers in favour, and only 283 against. A week later the *Sunday Mirror* reported the findings of a similar survey which found that twenty-four per cent of "young readers" agreed with the proposition that "Gays deserve Aids", with twenty-six per cent agreeing that "Anyone who sleeps around deserves Aids", and an overwhelming seventy-four per cent in favour of compulsory testing for everyone. But testing for *what*, and *by whom*, and *where*? When the Swedish government introduced compulsory testing for the sexual partners of anyone known to be HIV positive, doctors unsurprisingly refused point blank to carry out the tests. Yet another poll – and much the nastiest – appeared in the *News of The World* on 1 March. This found 56.8 per cent of readers in favour of the idea that "Aids carriers" should be "sterilised and given treatment to curb their sexual appetite", with a mere fifty-one per cent in favour of the total recriminalisation of homosexuality.

In point of fact the most recent evidence strongly suggests that, far from being the "cause" of Aids, gay men were routinely injected with HIV infected blood products, in the form of gamma globulin used in the treatment of hepatitis-B, which was prepared throughout the 1970s from blood which had been illegally imported from central Africa.[4] Fortunately the Minister of Health, Mr Norman Fowler, has recently rejected the notion of compulsory testing out of hand.[5] Nonetheless there remains the real possibility that limited mandatory testing might still be introduced for reasons of political expediency, as they have been in more than twelve other countries so far. It should by now be clear that the entire subject of HIV antibody testing, wilfully misinterpreted as "Aids testing", reflects an entirely *non-medical* agenda, and is the latest and lowest strategy developed by bigots and moralists of all persuasions to turn this terrible human tragedy to their own repugnant and sickening purposes. How else can one possibly explain the kind of agenda-setting implicit in the questions asked by the *Sunday Mirror* and the *News of The World*, which positively rejoice and celebrate in appalling human misery? Unfortunately, the BBC has already shown itself able and willing to follow this shocking lead, with a poll of its own asking whether testing should be compulsory, with a thoroughly predictable fifty-seven per cent of viewers (which ones?) supposedly in favour (*The AIDS Debate*, BBC1, 27 February). Any day now we can expect the press to catch up another stage with their American counterparts, with cynical calls for quarantine "on behalf" of PWAs themselves.

The recent television explosion concerning Aids has been much more uneven than one might have expected – both for better and for worse. It has also had its moments of high comedy, like the spectacle of Ian Dury tugging a condom down a fifteen-inch long white plastic phallus. Unfortunately, the same programme – *AIDS – The Facts*

(BBC1, 27 February) – introduced our old friend "the Aids virus", and found itself incapable of talking about gay men, preferring the pathologising discourse of "the homosexual". It also made the familiar and unhelpful distinction between the supposedly friable rectum and the tough, sturdy, trustworthy vagina. Since there is no evidence that vaginal sex with an infected partner is intrinsically safer than anal sex, the distinction, which has run right through British current affairs analysis, reveals a subtle skewing of how we think about sex which has nothing to do with actual risk factors. Dury also claimed, quite incorrectly, that Aids is always fatal "within a few weeks or months", which is a profoundly unhelpful observation for people struggling to come to terms with a recent diagnosis, and a matter for astonishment on the part of the many, many PWAs living full and productive lives in their first, second, or even third year of Aids. *AIDS – The Facts* ended with the singularly unfactual comment that, "You don't just catch Aids – you allow someone to give it to you." Whilst the intention here was clear, the means of conveying it was regrettable since, yet again, it suggests that it is Aids which is infectious, rather than HIV, thus making the lives of People With Aids that much more difficult since they are perceived as threatening rather than threatened.

Earlier in the same evening ITV offered us *First AIDS*, a programme aimed at young people, with a panel of ageing "experts" in front of a studio audience which was exclusively white and, as far as we ever learned, equally exclusively heterosexual. This was a surprising and very regrettable absence, since young lesbians and gays have so much that their straight contemporaries can learn from in terms of sexual maturity and articulateness. Gay teenagers are also, of course, far more at risk of HIV infection than other groups of young people. Nonetheless the programme did acknowledge the diversity of sexuality in a fairly non-judgemental way – even if it couldn't find its way to include a few smart young perverts. It also managed to tackle the difficult and important issue of embarrassment about buying condoms at the chemists, with a splendid interview with a young woman describing the agonies young people go through at the counter.

Unfortunately, however, the whole programme then took a deep dive into the murkiest realms of instant sociobiology. We learned, for example, that young men are driven (literally) by "the male sex drive", whilst girls are "naturally" passive and romantic. The hero of the day was undoubtedly testosterone, in a hormonally determined picture of human sexuality and gender, which simply masculinised sex, whilst totally marginalising young women who might actually enjoy sex, as "randy" and unnatural. Girls are supposed to go for "fashionable celibacy" before the universal goal of marriage and motherhood. This was all deeply distasteful, and was brilliantly, if all too briefly, given the lie by one young woman who pointed out that, "You have to kiss a lot of frogs before you find your prince".

Later that same evening the BBC showed *The Aids Debate*, chaired by the painfully sincere Robert Kilroy-Silk, with a large studio audience. But at least a loathsome journalist from *Today* got put firmly in his place after launching the press agenda concerning compulsory testing, which was soundly criticised by Professor Michael Adler (who also finds it impossible to use the awful word "gay" it seems) and Norman Fowler, as well as Jonathan Grimshawe who really deserves a prize for consistently being the only intelligent spokesperson on behalf of PWAs and HIV on British television. He had much to put up with from other speakers and, as I have described, a BBC poll concerning compulsory testing which was completely inexcusable, and a grim sign of the ways in which "popular" television feels obliged to imitate the very worst aspects of the tabloids. The best thing on the show was undoubtedly the mother of a PWA in the audience, Terry, and her few words were amongst the most moving and powerful – because so unrehearsed and understated and above all good humoured – of any heard on British television about Aids since 1983.

Predictably, a whole host of current affairs format programmes made sure that we didn't hear anything from such dangerous and contaminated sources. Indeed, the entire current affairs approach to Aids seems consistently determined at any cost to prevent viewers from making a positive identification of any kind with PWAs who are tacitly held to occupy a "guilty victim" status – unless, that is, they are prepared to act out the "guilty victim" role in what they say – as in last year's uniquely disgusting *Diverse Reports* production for Channel Four, *AIDS is A Four Letter Word*, and a host of other such productions. It is precisely this total inability to acknowledge the actual sexual diversity of the real viewing public which is currently being partially exposed at least on the better Aids programmes, amongst which was a series of ten minute long shorts which followed the *Ten O'clock News* on ITV. *AIDS Help* was presented by the *excellent* Viv Gee, who is far and away the best presenter of any Aids programme to date – confident, cheerful, and encouraging, in the face of so much counter-productive fatalism and gloom. The speakers on *AIDS Help* were uniformly well chosen and the short introductory fiction scenarios were models of their kind – well written, perfectly cast and acted.

Diametrically opposite to this approach was the BBC's nightly phone-in *AIDS Special*, hosted by the frequently flustered Patty

Caldwell, who was clearly out of her depth. The whole phone-in agenda on Aids colludes with tabloid journalism at its very considerable and formidable worst – as was apparent from Jonathan Dimbleby's recent and profoundly nauseating edition of *This Week* (23 October, 1986). It would appear that the BBC learned nothing from that lamentable precedent since they blithely proceeded with a series which, in the name of "public opinion", simply fanned the flames of ignorance, fear, bigotry and sexual paranoia. Thus on 4 March, for example, the *AIDS Special* on the subject of morality managed to imply that only Christians can define moral positions, in a dialogue between various born-again homophobes and a panel of experts which ranged from a liberal priest to one Dr Michael Ellis, with Nick Partridge from The Terrence Higgins Trust, who at least managed to slip in some eminently sensible words about the realities of sexual diversity in between the furious diatribes of phoned-in hatred and homophobia. Unfortunately, however, the "experts" were quite unable to match the passionately self-righteous shrieks of opinionated ignorance which swilled from the telephones.

It was left to Jeffrey Dickens M.P. to describe his forthcoming Private Member's Bill which aims to recriminalise homosexuality.[6] That this proposed legislation is entirely motivated by a homophobia which has nothing to do with its stated aim to control the spread of Aids is clear from its aim to criminalise lesbianism for the first time in British history. The fact that not one single voice has been raised in public to challenge the picture which Mr Dickens calmly described of a police force empowered to enter homes and break up gay relationships is a chilling reflection on the relentless miniaturisation of public considerations of the meaning of democracy in con- temporary Britain. It is this same climate which recently permitted the editor of the widely respected magazine *New Society* to defend his decision to publish a uniquely poisonous article by the predictably despicable Julie Burchill on the grounds that "gays" know what censorship is all about, and shouldn't expect it of him.

Ms Burchill had written an almost touchingly ignorant article,[7] in which she argued a doubly racist and homophobic case according to which all gay men are supposedly paedophile child-molesters, who have deservedly collectively contracted HIV as the revenge of The Dark Continent. To confuse responsible editorial policy with censorship is precisely the line of defence one has come to expect from the editor of the *Sun*, but not from *New Society*. Ms Burchill's baleful influence may be felt throughout British pop journalism, though it remains strongest in her original *alma mater The Face*.[8] Of her own literary performance I could say many things, but will confine myself (with difficulty) to Thackeray's description of Mr Osborne in *Vanity*

Fair – which might equally apply to most of the journalists, editors, script-writers and television presenters whose mighty contributions to our deeper understanding of Aids I've already mentioned: "He firmly believed," wrote Thackeray, "that everything he did was right, that he ought on all occasions to have his own way – and like the sting of a wasp or serpent his hatred rushed out armed and poisonous against anything like opposition. He was proud of his hatred as of everything else. Always to be right, always to trample forward, and never to doubt, are not these the great qualities with which dullness takes the lead in the world?"

Speaking at the annual Human Rights Campaign Fund dinner in New York, Coretta Scott King recently emphasised the point that she considers the movements for gay rights to be an integral part of the overall civil rights movement:

> "I am here tonight to express my solidarity with the gay and lesbian community in your struggle for civil and human rights in America and around the world. I believe all Americans who believe in freedom, tolerance and human rights have a responsibility to oppose bigotry and prejudice based on sexual orientation."[9]

Here in Britain the fact must be faced that nobody of Coretta King's stature exists to speak such words. No major public institutions exist at which such words might be spoken. And no political tradition exists which might record, let alone heed them. This is our tragedy – the measure of our ethical bankruptcy as a nation, and the moral bankruptcy of our entire political system.

For the last five years everyone working in the broad arena of Aids work has had to contend with the consequences of total government inaction and a media campaign of unequalled viciousness against people with Aids, their friends, loved ones, and families. The television and newspaper industries have laboriously constructed a punitive palisade around the entire subject which guarantees that Aids is still popularly thought of as a self-inflicted condition, and an index of moral turpitude. Onto this hideous landscape the government has now directed a nationwide leaflet-drop and media campaign which has done nothing to challenge those assumptions, and subtly colludes with them. The densely impacted sexual guilt and ignorance of an entire culture is now being expressed in a displaced form as anxiety about Aids. In this manner a personalised moral agenda for thinking about Aids is also being orchestrated into actual social policy. Government ministers have already stated their intention to proceed with legislation to prevent what they understand as the "promotion" of homosexuality and

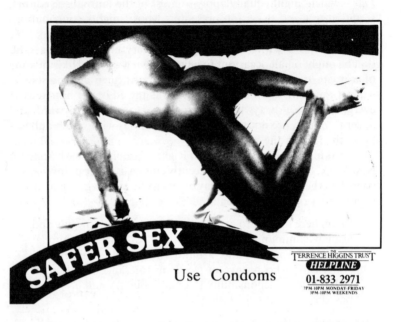

lesbianism, which the minister of local government Dr Rhodes Boyson has justified as necessary to protect the survival of the species.[10] It is critically important to recognise that Aids can now be used to "justify" any amount of conservative legislation concerning sexuality, with a high proportion of active popular consent. This is why debates about censorship matter in a wholly new way. It is thus especially regrettable that, for example, the National Council for Civil Liberties should be calling for increased legal restrictions on the representation of sexuality at this of all times, on the misguided and totally misleading model of anti-racist laws.[11] Whether we like it or not, debates about sexuality and representation are now at the very heart of British and American politics, and the political imagination of our times.

The appointment of newspaper magnate Robert Maxwell as the leading fund-raiser for a government-backed charitable trust to support the hospice movement and medical research suggests that Aids is also regarded as a precedent to allow the sweeping aside of all previous values and working practices of socialised medicine in the United Kingdom. News that the Bloomsbury district health authority in central London cannot afford to supply the drug AZT to the 120 people with Aids in its care is as unpardonable as it is unprecedented.

This is thought to be "the first time that such an approved drug has been officially withheld from National Health Service patients on financial grounds".[12] Although adequate funding has now been made available, the situation of the person with Aids who had been denied the only drug which is currently able to prevent the HIV virus from reproducing itself within the blood does not bear much contemplation. This story, which first emerged in the gay press, was turned down by several national daily newspapers, and only finally appeared in the *Guardian* after two weeks had passed by. In such circumstances the radical instability and unevenness of Aids commentary continues casually to countenance the gravest infringements of fundamental human rights and dignities.

Thus on the same day in May 1987 the *Sun* offered free one-way airline tickets to Norway in order to encourage gay men to leave Britain for good, under the headline "Fly away gays – and we will pay!"[13] whilst the *Guardian* cynically framed the diary of a positively identified gay man with Aids with the headline "The diary of a condemned man".[14] This was particularly regrettable since the diary in question had been written by a man who had only gradually come to accept his homosexuality in his late thirties, after years of guilt and repression. He is brave, and above all optimistic – the very antithesis of the fatalistic doomladen imagery which the *Guardian* foisted on him. Not content with having privileged the connotations of the condemned cell as the "correct" way to think about Aids, an accompanying photograph was printed showing a group of men holding up a banner announcing them as members of the "People With Aids Alliance". This was accompanied by an astonishingly insensitive text which read: "Immunised against embarrassment: American Aids victims". Aids is evidently still such an embarrassing subject for most journalists that they will stop at nothing to compass and confine the experience of people with Aids in their own insultingly victimising terms. It is clear that whatever gay men write in newspapers or say on television will be skewed in advance to the interests and values of an entirely fictive general public. That is why we must refuse, absolutely, to inhabit the immensely convenient role of the "victim", which has been so generously dug to contain us like a mass grave. As James Baldwin has noted:

> "The victim can have no point of view for precisely as long as he thinks of himself as a victim. The testimony of the victim, as victim, corroborates, simply, the reality of the chains that bind him – confirms, and, as it were, consoles the jailer, the keeper of the keys. For precisely as long as the jailer hears your moaning, he knows where you are. The sound of the

victim's moaning confirms the authority of the jailer, the keeper of the keys: those keys that, designed to lock you out, inexorably lock him in. He is the prisoner of the delusion of his power, to which he has surrendered any possibility of identity, or the private life, and he glimpses this, sometimes, in his mirror, or in the eyes of his children. His only real hope is death. That is why he cannot love his children, the proof being that he dare not consider his dreadful legacy, this fire-bombed earth: his only real achievement".[15]

At this moment in time it is therefore up to lesbians and gay men to expose the disgusting "morality" which calmly proclaims that Aids is the just deserts for all those who have had sex outside marriage in the last ten years – which is the indisputable explanation of British and American governmental policy these last five years and more. The true measure of our societies' respective capacities for self-deception lies in their piteous dependence on a myth of the family – a myth which, like all other myths, "deals in false universals, to dull the pain of particular circumstances", as Angela Carter explains.[10] Homosexuality will only continue to confront this culture with an unbearable degree of pain as long as it continues to subscribe to this laughably inadequate sacramental model for envisaging and evaluating *all* forms of human social, sexual and erotic relationships and pleasures. It is a myth which fails miserably to do justice either to the actualities of parenting, or to any of the multitude of sexual and erotic bonds which exist independently of child-bearing, for women and men and young people alike.

In this, as in every other respect, the media's response to Aids is transparently defensive, its raving like that of the red-faced playground bully who suddenly finds himself alone and confronted by a quiet organised crowd which refuses to be bullied any more. For Aids affects a generation of gay men which has already long ago refused to accept second class citizenship, even if that refusal has not yet found coherent political or institutional expression. We know with Whitman that "one is no better than the other". We know that if our species has any worth or beauty it lies in its diversity, and our capacity to embrace and celebrate all our variously consenting states of desire. And if in these terrible times we should wish somewhat to alleviate the pain of our losses – of freedoms and of friends – then we might think of Aids as a monstrously ironic means to this end, and of our loved ones who have died as martyrs to that great cause.

Notes

Introduction
1. The *Observer*, 5 October, 1986.
2. Richard Goldstein, "A Plague On All Our Houses", the *Village Voice*, vol. xxxi, no. 36, 16 September, 1986.
3. Julia Neuberger, "Aids and the cruelty of panic", The *Guardian*, 9 December, 1985.
4. Simon Watney, "The Rhetoric of AIDS", *Screen*, vol. 27, no. 1, January–February, 1986.
5. David M. Lowe, "Where Do We Go From Here?", the *Sentinel* (San Francisco), vol. 14, no. 16, 1 August, 1986.
6. Ibid.

Chapter One: Sex, diversity and disease
1. Iris Murdoch, *The Fire And The Sun*, Oxford, 1976, p. 87.
2. Jeffrey Weeks, *Sexuality and its Discontents: Meanings, Myths & Modern Sexualities*, R.K.P., 1985, p. 45.
3. Richard Dyer, "The Celluloid Closet", *Birmingham Arts Lab. Bulletin*, 1 April – 30 June, 1982, p. 43
4. Allan Barratt, "Saving Sex", *New York Native*, issue 161, 19 May, 1986.
5. Jacqueline Rose, *The Case Of Peter Pan, or The Impossibility of Children's Fiction*, Macmillan, 1984, p. 16.
6. Allan M. Brandt, *No Magic Bullet: A Social History of Venereal Disease in The United States Since 1880*, Oxford University Press, 1987, p. 202.
7. Ibid., p. 203.
8. Larry Kramer, "1,112 And Counting", *New York Native*, issue 59, 14–27 March, 1983.
9. Richard Goldstein, "Heartsick: Fear and Loving in the Gay Community", *Village Voice*, vol. xxvii, no. 26, 28 June, 1983.
10. Ibid.
11. The *Guardian*, 15 March, 1986.
12. Dennis Altman, *The Homosexualisation of America*, Beacon Press, 1982, p. xi.
13. Michel Foucault, *Discipline and Punish*, Peregrine, 1979, pp. 25–26.
14. Dennis Altman, op. cit., p. 188.
15. See Michel Foucault, "Power and Sex", *Telos*, no. 32, 1977.
16. Carole S. Vance, "The Meese Commission on The Road", *The Nation*, 2–9 August, 1986.
17. Casey L. Klinger, *Jock*, January, 1986.
18. See Rick Bebout and Doug Grenville, "No More Shit", *The Body Politic*, no. 127, June, 1986.
19. Michel Halberstadt, "The Argot of Dreams" *New York Native*, issue 167, 30 June, 1986.
20. Wayne C. Olson, "Transcending Gayness", *New York Native*, issue 160, 12 May, 1986.
21. Joseph Puccia, "Going Underground", *New York Native*, issue 160, 12 May, 1986.
22. Jeffrey Weeks, *Sexuality*, Tavistock, 1986, p. 73.
23. Ibid., p. 24.

Chapter Two: Infectious desires

1. Gayle Rubin, "Thinking Sex: Notes for a Radical Theory of the Politics of Sexuality", in *Pleasure and Danger: Exploring Female Sexuality*, Carole S. Vance (Ed.), R.K.P., 1984, p. 267.
2. Maurice Blanchot, *The Writing of The Disaster*, University of Nebraska Press, 1986, p. 66.
3. Dr Jonathan Rodney, *A Handbook of Sex Knowledge*, Paul Elek, 1961, p. 107.
4. Simon Watney, "On Gay Liberation", *Politics & Power* no. 4, RKP, 1981, p. 300.
5. Edmund White, *A Boy's Own Story*, Dutton, 1982, p. 126.
6. See Simon Watney, "Katharine Hepburn and The Cinema of Chastisement", *Screen*, vol. 26, no. 5, 1985.
7. See J. Laplanche and J.-B. Pontalis, *The Language of Psycho-Analysis*, Hogarth Press, 1983, p. 277.
8. Neil Bartlett, "Designs for Living", *The Body Politic*, no. 125, April, 1986.
9. The *Sunday Times*, 24 August, 1986, p. 39.
10. *The Nine O'Clock News*, BBC1, 8 August, 1986.
11. *Working Woman*, September, 1986.
12. James Baldwin, *The Devil Finds Work*, Michael Joseph, 1978.

Chapter Three: Mortal panics

1. *The Letters of Sylvia Townsend Warner*, W. Maxwell (Ed.), Chatto & Windus, 1982, p. 73.
2. Peg Byron, "No Room At The Ward: City Hospitals Hide from Aids", the *Village Voice*, 20 May, 1986, p. 27.
3. *Capital Gay*, no. 203, 2 August, 1985.
4. *Daily Mirror*, 19 February, 1985.
5. Stanley Cohen, *Folk Devils and Moral Panics: The Creation of The Mods And Rockers (1972)*, Martin Robertson, 1980, p. 9.
6. Ibid., p. 17.
7. Ibid, p. 154.
8. Ibid, p. 154.
9. Stuart Hall et. al. (Eds.), *Policing the Crisis*, Macmillan, 1978, p. 221.
10. Jeffrey Weeks, *Sexuality and Its Discontents: Meanings, Myths, & Modern Sexualities*, R.K.P., 1985, p. 45.
11. Gayle Rubin, "Thinking Sex: Notes for a Radical Theory of the Politics of Sexuality", in *Pleasure and Danger: Exploring Female Sexuality*, Carole S. Vance (Ed.), R.K.P., 1984, p. 297.
12. Dennis Altman, *Aids And The New Puritanism*, Pluto, 1986, p. 186.
13. Ibid., p. 187.
14. The *Guardian*, 16 July, 1986.
15. William F. Buckley, "Identify All The Carriers", The *New York Times*, 18 March, 1986, p. A27.
16. Alan M. Dershowitz, "Emphasize Scientific Information", The *New York Times*, 18 March, 1986, p. A27.
17. Digby Anderson, "No moral panic – that's the problem", the *Times*, 18 March, 1985.
18. Eric Eckholm, "Study of Aids Victims Families Doubts Disease Is Transmitted Casually", the *New York Times*, 6 February, 1986, p. 87.
19. Dr George Weinberg, *Society and the Healthy Homosexual*, Doubleday Anchor, 1973, p. xi.
20. See Louis Crompton, *Byron & Greek Love*, Faber & Faber, 1985. Also, Simon Watney, "Paralyzing Posterity", *London Review of Books*, vol. 7, no. 14, 1 August, 1985, p. 4.
21. James Naughtie, "Minister blames gays for Spread of Aids", the *Guardian*, 5 September, 1985.
22. Enrique Rueda, *The Homosexual Network*, USA, 1983.

23. See Simon Watney, "The Banality of Gender", *Oxford Literary Review*, vol. 8, nos. 1–2, 1986.
24. See J. Laplanche and J.-B. Pontalis, *The Language of Psycho-Analysis*, Hogarth Press, 1983, p. 376.
25. Ibid., p. 378.
26. Sigmund Freud, "The Unconscious", in *On Metapsychology: The Theory of Psychoanalysis*, Pelican Freud Library, vol. 11, 1984, p. 187.
27. Joe Baker, "Inside Anita's Ministries of Guilt", *The Advocate*, issue 265, 19 April, 1979.
28. Quoted in Ann Guidici Fettner, "The Evil That Men Do", *New York Native*, issue 127, 23–29 September, 1985.
29. *New York Native,* issue 167, 30 June, 1986.
30. Glenn Wilson, *Love And Instinct*, Temple Smith, 1982.
31. See Andrea Dworkin, *Pornography*, The Women's Press, 1983.
32. Glenn Wilson, op. cit.
33. Michael Neve, "Animal Crackers", *London Review of Books*, vol. 8, no. 9, 22 May, 1986.
34. *New York Native*, issue 156, 14 April, 1986.
35. *Obscene Publications (Protection of Children, Etc.) (Amendment) Bill*, 4 December, 1985, Her Majesty's Stationery Office.
36. Dr Joseph Sonnabend, "Looking at Aids in Totality: A Conversation", *New York Native*, issue 129, 7–13 October, 1985.
37. *BBC News*, Radio Four, 11 September, 1986.
38. See Leeds Revolutionary Feminist Group, *Love Your Enemy?*, Onlywomen Press, 1981, which is discussed at length by Susan Ardill and Sue O'Sullivan, "Upsetting The Applecart: Difference, Desire, and Lesbian Sadomasochism", *Feminist Review*, no. 23, summer, 1986

Chapter Four: Aids, pornography and law

1. Paul Hirst, "Law and Sexual Difference", *Oxford Literary Review*, vol. 8, nos. 1–2, 1986, p. 193.
2. *Capital Gay*, no. 245, 6 June, 1986.
3. Donna Turley, "The Feminist Debate on Pornography", *Socialist Review*, no. 87–88, May–August, 1986.
4. Carole S. Vance, "The Meese Commission On The Road", *The Nation*, 2–9 August, 1986.
5. Beverley Brown, "Private faces in public spaces", *Ideology & Consciousness*, no. 7, 1980, p. 3.
6. Jeffrey Weekes, *Sexuality And Its Discontents: Meanings, Myths and Modern Sexualities*, R.K.P., 1985, p. 54.
7. Ibid., p. 55.
8. Donna Turley, op. cit., p. 87.
9. Ibid., p. 89.
10. Jeffrey Weeks, *Sex, Politics and Society: The regulation of sexuality since 1800*, Longmans, 1981, p. 42.
11. Ibid., p. 81.
12. Richard Summerhill, "Porn Crime", *The Body Politic*, no. 109, December, 1984.
13. T. R. Witomski, "The 'Sickness' of Pornography", *New York Native*, issue 121, 29 July – 11 August, 1985.
14. Chris Bearchell, "Pornography, Prostitution and Moral Panic", *The Body Politic*, no. 101, March, 1984.
15. Paul Crane, *Gays and The Law*, Pluto Press, 1983, p. 87.
16. Annette Kuhn, "Public versus private: the case of indecency and obscenity", *Leisure Studies*, no. 3, 1984, p. 53.
17. Ibid., p. 59.
18. Chris Smith, *Capital Gay*, 4 July, 1986.

19. Jo Richardson, reported in *Gay Times*, no. 89, February, 1986.
20. Gayle Rubin, "Thinking Sex: Notes for a Radical Theory of the Politics of Sexuality", in *Pleasure and Danger: Exploring Female Sexuality*, Carole S. Vance (Ed.), R.K.P., 1984, p. 271.
21. *Gay Times*, no. 95, August, 1986.
22. Carole S. Vance, op. cit. (1986), p. 77.
23. Ibid., p. 78.
24. The *Guardian*, 29 July, 1986.
25. Laura Cottingham, "Anti-Porn and Its Discontents", *New York Native*, 3–16 December, 1984.
26. Angela Carter, "The Language of Sisterhood", in *The State Of The Language*, L. Michaels and C. Ricks (Eds.), California, 1980.
27. Susanne Kappeler, "Censored: The Porn Debate", *New Socialist*, no. 36, March, 1986.
28. Rosalind Coward, "What's In It For Women?", *New Statesman*, 13 June, 1986.
29. Beverley Brown, "A Feminist Interest in Pornography – Some Modest Proposals", *m/f* nos. 5–6, 1981, p. 5.
30. Ibid.
31. Ibid., p. 11.
32. Simon Watney, "Porno-babble", *New Socialist*, no. 39, June, 1986.
33. Letter to *New York Native*, issue 137, 2 – 9 December, 1985.
34. T. R. Witomski, op. cit.

Chapter Five: Aids and the press
1. Neil R. Schram, "AIDS: 1991", *Los Angeles Times Magazine*, vol. 11, no. 32, 10 August, 1986.
2. Charles Linebarger, "LaRouche Prop Hit On \$7–20 Billion Cost", *Bay Area Reporter*, vol. xvi, no. 33, 14 August, 1986.
3. *New York Native*, issue 168, 7 July, 1986.
4. Martin Amies, "Making Sense of Aids", the *Observer*, 23 June, 1985.
5. Ibid.
6. Leo Bersani, *Baudelaire and Freud*, California, 1977, p. 129.
7. "Panic", *The Face*, no. 61, May, 1985.
8. J. Laplanche and J.-B. Pontalis, *The Language of Psycho-Analysis*, Hogarth Press, 1973, pp. 118–119.
9. George Gordon, "Haunted by the Epidemic of Fear", *Daily Mail*, 3 October, 1986.
10. J. Laplanche and J.-B. Pontalis, op. cit., p. 194.
11. The *Sun*, 30 August, 1983.
12. Anthony Doran, "Such a gay day down Lambeth way", *Daily Mail*, 31 May, 1985.
13. The *Star*, 3 July, 1986.
14. Kevin O'Sullivan, "It's Eastbenders", the *Sun*, 13 August, 1986.
15. Baz Bamigboye and Peter McKay, "The Last Days of Rock Hudson", *Daily Mail*, 3 October, 1985.
16. Charles Catchpole, "The Hunk Who Lived a Lie", the *Sun*, 3 October, 1985.
17. Paul Callan, "Rock, A Soul in Torment", the *Mirror*, 3 October, 1985.
18. Tony Brooks, "The Heart-Throb Who Lived a Lie", the *Star*, 3 October, 1985.
19. Terry Willows, the *Star*, 5 August, 1985.
20. Michel Foucault, "Sexual Choice, Sexual Act: An Interview", *Salmagundi*, nos. 58–59, fall/winter, 1982/83.
21. *Daily Mail*, 27 December, 1985.
22. The *Sun*, 3 October, 1985 (photographer, Phillip Ramey).
23. The *Standard*, 3 October, 1985.
24. Nick Ferran, "Madonna Buys Rock's Plague Palace", the *Sun*, 2 September, 1986.
25. Baz Bamigboye and Peter McKay, op. cit.

26. *Daily Free-Lance*, Henryetta, Oklahoma, 3 October, 1985.
27. Frances FitzGerald, "A Reporter At Large (San Francisco – Part 2)", *The New Yorker*, vol. LX11, no. 23, 28 July, 1986, p. 49.
28. Edmund White, "Aids: An American Epidemic", afterword to *States of Desire* (1980), Picador, 1986, pp. 341–2.
29. James F. Grutsch and A. D. J. Robertson, "The Coming of AIDS", *The American Spectator*, March, 1986.
30. Duncan Fallowell, the *Times*, 27 July, 1983.
31. Birstol Watershed, 2 August, 1986.
32. Robin McKie, the *Observer*, 3 August, 1986.
33. Simon Kinnersley, "This baby's got AIDS!", *Woman's Own*, 3 May, 1986.
34. Simon Kinnersley, "The sad sad story of the woman with AIDS", *Woman's Own*, 12 July, 1986.
35. Peter Cliff, "My Misery Posing as AIDS Victim", the *Sun*, 23 January, 1986.
36. John Lisners, "I'd Shoot My Son If He Had AIDS, Says Vicar", the *Sun*, 14 October, 1985.
37. J. Laplanche and J.-B. Pontalis, op. cit., p. 398.
38. John Marshall, "Press Council Rejects Complaint Against The Sun", *Gay Times*, no. 92, May, 1986.
39. Alfred Kazin, "In Washington", *New York Review of Books*, vol. xxxiii, no. 9, 29 May, 1986, p. 18.
40. Nicholas de Jongh, "When the Real Disease is press distortion", the *Guardian*, 14 April, 1986.
41. Ibid.

Chapter Six: Aids on television
1. *Are We Being Served*, The London Media Project, 1986.
2. James Curran and Jean Seaton, *Power Without Responsibility: The Press And Broadcasting in Britain*, Methuen, 1985, p. 179.
3. Mandy Merck, "'Gay Life': Desire, Demography And Disappointment", *Gay Left*, no. 10, 1980, p. 16.
4. *Where There's Life*, ITV, 15 August, 1986.
5. Professor Michael Adler, letter to the *Guardian*, 14 August, 1986.
6. Stuart Hall, "The rediscovery of 'ideology': the return of the repressed in media studies", in *Culture, Society and The Media*, M. Gurevitch et al. (Eds.), Methuen, 1982, p. 76.
7. "AIDS: A Strange and Deadly Virus", BBC *Horizon*, 24 March, 1986.
8. Stephen Farber, "A Drama of Family Loyalty, Acceptance – and AIDS", *New York Times*, 1985.
9. See Simon Watney, "Hollywood's Homosexual World", *Screen*, vol. 23, nos. 3–4, 1982.
10. Darrell Yates Rist, "Fear and Loving and AIDS", *Film Comment*, April, 1986.
11. *Buddies*, Channel Four, 15 September, 1986.
12. Darrell Yates Rist, op. cit.
13. "AIDS is a four-letter word", *Diverse Reports* for Channel Four, 17 September, 1986.
14. The *Guardian*, 11 August, 1986.
15. Peter Tatchell, letter to the *Guardian*, 14 August, 1986.
16. "Saint Genet", BBC2 *Arena*, 3 May, 1986.

Chapter Seven: Safer representations
1. Edmund White, "Interview: A Testing Dilemma", *Gay Times*, no. 93, June, 1986.
2. Stuart Hall, "The rediscovery of 'ideology': return of the repressed in media studies", in *Culture, Society And The Media*, M. Gurevitch et al. (Eds.), Methuen, 1982, p. 64.
3. Ellen Willis, "Feminism, Moralism and Pornography", in *Desire: The Politics of Sexuality*, Ann Snitow et al. (Eds.), Virago, 1984, pp. 84–5.

4. Michel Foucault, "On Governmentality", *Ideology & Consciousness*, no. 6, autumn, 1979, p. 17.
5. Kaye Wellings, *Sickness And Sin, The Case of Genital Herpes*, paper presented to BSA Medical Sociology Group, 1983, p. 10.
6. Ibid., p. 26.
7. Robert Glück, *Jack The Modernist*, Gay Presses of New York, p. 54.
8. W. H. Auden, *Horae Canonicae*.
9. Andrew Lesk, "MD diagnosed with bias", *The Body Politic*, no. 125, April, 1986.
10. Joy Melville, "First Aids", the *Guardian*, 24 September, 1986.
11. Professor Anthony Pinching, letter to the *Guardian*, 22 September, 1986.
12. R. Gittings (Ed.), *The Letters Of John Keats*, Oxford, 1975, pp. 391–2.
13. John Preston (Ed.), *Hot Living: Erotic Stories About Safer Sex*, Alyson Publications, 1985.
14. Jonathan Hales, "AIDS: The Youth View", *Gay Times*, no. 95, August, 1986.
15. J. Laplanche and J.-B. Pontalis, "Fantasy and The Origins of Sexuality", *The International Journal Of Psycho-Analysis*, vol. 49, 1968.
16. Adam Carr, "Safe Sex: Can You Keep It Up?" *Mister*, no. 51, 1985 (reprinted from *Outrage*, Australia).
17. J. McLaren, "Europe gets safe sex parties", *Capital Gay*, 17 January, 1986.
18. Peg Byron, "AIDS Education: The City's Closet Case", the *Village Voice*, 28 May, 1985, p. 33.
19. Ann Guidici Fettner, "Is The CDC Dying of Aids?", *Village Voice*, vol. xxxi, no. 40, 7 October, 1986.
20. Thucydides, *History Of The Peloponnesian War*, Penguin, 1972, p. 155.

Epilogue
1. John Carvell, "Cabinet Aids Drive aimed at all homes", the *Guardian*, 12 November, 1986.
2. Nicholas Timmins, "Aids numbers climb steadily", the *Independent*, 10 March, 1987.
3. Oliver Gillie, "Arson attacks on homes of Aids victims", the *Independent*, 2 February, 1987.
4. Larry Kramer, "Dr Mathilde Krim", *Interview Magazine*, Vol. XVII, No. 2, February, 1987. See also Andrew Veitch, "The Spread of Aids blamed on blood trade", the *Guardian*, 22 March, 1985.
5. *The AIDS Debate*, BBC1, 27 February, 1987.
6. *Heart Of The Matter*, BBC1, 8 March, 1987.
7. Julie Burchill, "Personal Piece", *New Society*, 20 February, 1987.
8. See, for example, William Leith, "Flirting", *i-D* Magazine, No. 44, February, 1987, and articles by Ian Penman and Marek Kohn in *The Face*, No. 83, March, 1987.
9. Peter Freiberg, "Coretta Scott King addresses HRCF", *The Advocate*, Issue 459, 11 November, 1986.
10. John Williams, "Government plans a blitz on gays", the *Evening Standard*, 8 May, 1987.
11. See Barbara Rogers' interview with Cathy Itzin from NCCL, "Pornography Incites Hatred", *Everywoman*, No. 27, May, 1987.
12. Andrew Veitch, "Cash-starved authority stops buying Aids drug", the *Guardian*, 13 May, 1987.
13. The *Sun*, 6 May, 1987.
14. Chris Dale, "The diary of a condemned man", the *Guardian*, 6 May, 1987.
15. James Baldwin, *The Evidence Of Things Not Seen*, Holt & Co. (USA), 1986, p. 78.
16. Angela Carter, *The Sadeian Woman: An Exercise in Cultural History*, Virago, 1978, p. 5.

Suggestions for further reading

Although bookshop shelves are groaning under the weight of books about Aids, most of these do not need to have the dust blown off. One exception is Dennis Altman's *AIDS And The New Puritanism* (Pluto Press, 1986), which examines the American context of Aids organisations and funding with considerable acuity. Although he has been accused of timidity, and of distancing himself from the epidemic, such charges only ultimately represent naive wishes for instant emotional answers to extremely complex social and economic problems. The most recent edition of *No Magic Bullet: A Social History of Veneral Disease in The United States Since 1880* by Allan M. Brandt contains an excellent chapter on Aids (Oxford University Press, 1987). The work of Leo Bersani offers the most intelligent commentary of which I am aware on the operations of fantasy within the field of cultural production. Newcomers to psychoanalytic theory might well begin with his *Baudelaire And Freud* (University of California, 1977). Mark Cousins and Athar Hussain have written the most perceptive study of the work of *Michel Foucault*, in a book of the same name (Macmillan, 1984), and of Foucault's own writings I am obliged to recommend *The History Of Sexuality: An Introduction* (Vintage Books, 1978) which is the *locus classicus* for all subsequent debate in this area. *The Birth Of The Clinic* (Tavistock, 1973) also offers an indispensible account of the emergence of the modern forms of medico-political power. Foucault's colleague Jaques Donzelot has written an equally seminal text about the forms of modern power and governmentality in *The Policing Of Families: Welfare versus the State* (Hutchinson, 1979).

Powers Of Horror: An Essay on Abjection (Columbia, 1982), by Julia Kristeva, provides an extremely stimulating series of meditations on the subject of the human body, death, and the sanitisation of subjectivity, although lesbian and gay readers should be on the alert for a subtle but pervasive current of homophobia here, as in all her work. *Life and Death in Psycho-Analysis* (Johns Hopkins, 1976), by J. Laplanche, is a standard text on the diversity of sexuality, and should be read in consultation with *The Language of Psycho-Analysis*, which he co-authored with J.-B. Pontalis. Both books provide profound critical commentaries on the work of Sigmund Freud, the range of whose writings lies beyond the scope of these suggestions, although I would draw the reader's attention at least to Volume 10 of The Pelican Freud Library, *On Psychopathology*. Cindy Patton's *Sex and Germs: The Politics of AIDS* (South End Press, 1985) has only recently landed on my desk from the United States, too late for me to refer to it in this book, but it seems to be a perceptive and thoughtful survey of the climate surrounding Aids in contemporary America, and with Dennis Altman is head and shoulders above other available books on the subject.

Plagues And Peoples (Penguin, 1979), by William H. McNeill, examines the role of epidemic illnesses in human history, and complements Hans Zinsser's classic, *Rats, Lice & History: The Biography of a Bacillus (1934)*, lately reprinted by Macmillan, in 1985. From the torrent of books about pornography I would single out *Pleasure And Danger: Exploring Female Sexuality*, edited by Carole S. Vance, as the most politically and intellectually acute, to be matched perhaps with Toril Moi's *Sexual/Textual Politics* (Methuen, 1985), which in my experience offers the most lucid and accessible introduction to contemporary debates in French feminist theory. Her section on Julia Kristeva is particularly rewarding. Finally I reach the work of Jeffrey Weeks, whose latest book *Sexuality* (Tavistock, 1986) elegantly condenses at least a decade of thought and historical analysis on the subject of sex and sexual politics, providing new readers with a panoramic survey of issues – which they will need to consult, follow up and explore in his earlier books in the detail they deserve.

Index

Acheson, Dr Donald 119
Adler, Professor Michael 34, 104, 143
Advocate, The 13, 58, 128
AIDS – The Victims 105
Allen, Woody 98
Altman, Dennis 14, 17, 40, 41, 155, 156
American Spectator, The 91
An Early Frost 92, 113, 114
Anderson, Digby 45, 46
Athletic Model Guild 65
Auden, W. H. 130

Baldwin, James 37, 147
Bartlett, Neil 28
BBC 29, 31, 32, 36, 110, 122, 129, 141, 142, 143, 144
Bearchell, Chris 63
Bersani, Leo 155
Blanchot, Maurice 150
Body Politic, The 128
Boy George 43, 44
Boyson, Dr Rhodes 146
Brandt, Allan M. 10, 155
British Medical Journal 30, 31
Brookside 100
Brown, Beverley 60, 71, 72
Bryant, Anita 50
Buckley, William F. 44, 46
Buddies 114
Burchill, Julie 80, 144
Burdus, Ann 138
Byron, Peg 154

Cameron, Paul 55
Carter, Angela 70, 148
Centers for Disease Control (USA) 8, 43, 50, 140
Chapman, Christine 115, 116, 117, 118, 119, 120, 121

Churchill Amendment Bill (1986) 59, 67
Cliff, Peter 94, 140
Cohen, Stanley 39, 43
Conservative Family Campaign 55, 56
Cousins, Mark 155
Coward, Rosalind 70, 71
Crane, Paul 65
Crompton, Louis 150

Daily Mail 81, 82, 83, 88, 89, 90
Dannemeyer, William 55
Dawson, Dr John 30, 31
de Jongh, Nicholas 97
Dickens, Jeffrey 144
Dimbleby, Jonathan 144
Diverse Reports 120, 143
Donzelot, Jaques 155
Dury, Ian 141, 142
Dworkin, Andrea 52, 59, 61, 70
Dyer, Richard 8

EastEnders 87
Ellis, Dr Michael 144
Evening Standard 140

Face, The 80, 144
Falwell, Jerry 63
Family Planning Association 127
Farthing, Dr Charles 30, 31
Ferriman, Annabel 92
Fettner, Ann Guidici 135
Fitzgerald, Frances 90, 91
Fitzgerald, Scott 3
Foucault, Michel 16, 89, 123, 126, 155
Fowler, Norman 141, 143
Freud, Sigmund 21, 49, 50, 80, 95, 155

Gai Pied 17, 128
Gay Left 99
Gay Life 99, 108
Gay Men's Health Crisis 75, 135
Gay News 66
Gay Times 59, 96
Gay's The Word Bookshop 17, 58, 59, 66
Genet, Jean 17, 122
Glück, Robert 127
Goldstein, Richard 3
Gordon, George 81, 82, 83
Grimshawe, Jonathan 143
Guardian 55, 147

Halberstadt, Michael 19, 20
Hall, Stuart 40, 124
Hancock, Graham 119, 120
Hannah And Her Sisters 98
Heaven 107
Hegarty, Paul 59
Hirst, Paul 58
Horizon 110
Hudson, Rock 87, 88, 89, 90
Hussain, Athar 155

Jobey, Liz 29

Kappeler, Susanne 70, 71
Keats, John 132
Kilroy-Silk, Robert 143
King, Coretta Scott 145
Kinnersley, Simon 92, 93, 94
Kramer, Larry 11
Kristeva, Julia 155, 156
Kuhn, Annette 65

Labour Party 64, 67
Laplanche, J. 50, 81, 155
Larouche initiative (1986) 17, 78
Livingstone, Ken 83
London Media Project 98
London Portrait 38
London Weekend Television 99, 108
Los Angeles Times Magazine 77

McDonald, Boyd 17, 75
McKay, John 48, 49, 130
McKie, Robin 1, 2, 33, 34, 35, 36, 103, 104, 105
MacKinnon, Katherine 59, 70
MacLean, Charles 140
McNeill, William H. 156
Mason, Dr James 51
Maxwell, Robert 146
Medical News 131
Meldrum, Julian 108
Merck, Mandy 99, 100
Miller, David 102, 107
Mirror 88
Morgan, Robin 63
Murdoch, Iris 7
Murdoch, Rupert 15, 29, 138

Naked Civil Servant, The 100
Narayan, Professor Opendra 111, 112
National Council for Civil Liberties 146
National Union of Journalists 96,
Neuberger, Julia 3
New Socialist 70
New Society 144
New York Native 13, 17, 58, 75, 123, 128
New York Post 131
New York Times 46, 68
New Yorker, The 90
Newman, Sir Kenneth 69, 70
News Of The World 141
Normal Heart, The 115

Observer 1, 2, 92
Olson, Wayne C. 20, 21

Partridge, Nick 144
Patton, John 104
People 83
Pinching, Professor Anthony 1, 105, 130
Pontalis, J.-B. 50, 81, 155
Preston John 132
Puccia, Joseph 20, 21

Rist, Darrell Yates 113
Rogers, Dr Adrian 54, 56
Rolling Stone 54
Rose, Jacqueline 10
Rubin, Gayle 22, 40

Schatz, Ben 5
Seitzman, Dr Peter 38
Sexual Offences Act (1967) 60
Smith, Chris 66, 67, 109
Sonnabend, Dr Joseph 53, 68
Star 85
Stoppard, Dr Miriam 100, 101
Summerhill, Richard 62, 63
Sun 82, 88, 89, 90, 94, 95, 96, 107,
    109, 129, 140, 144
Sunday Mirror 141
Sunday Times 29

Tatchell, Peter 109, 121
Tedder, Dr Richard 102
Terrence Higgins Trust, The 94, 108,
    110, 118, 119, 130, 134, 144
Thackeray, W. M. 145
Thames Television 105
Thatcher, Margaret 15
This Week 144
Thucydides 135
Times 45, 91, 92
Today 143
Turley, Donna 61, 62

Union World 109

Vance, Carole S. 68, 69, 156
Village Voice 44

Wahl, John 5
Walden, Brian 102, 103, 104
Warner, Sylvia Townsend 38
Waugh, Evelyn 97
Weaver, Dr Jonathan 106
Weaver, Martin 119
Weber, Bruce 29
Weeks, Jeffrey 8, 21, 40, 62, 109, 156
Weiss, Professor Robin 116, 117
Wellings, Kaye, 127
West, Peter 104
Where There's Life 100, 101 ·
White, Edmund 17, 24, 90, 91, 123
Whitehouse, Mary 66, 121
Whitman, Walt 148
Wilde, Oscar 17
Williams, Tennessee 17
Wilson, Glenn 51, 52
Withington, John 38
Wodehouse, Pandora 32
Wolfenden Report (1957) 60
Wolfenden Strategy 60, 61, 64, 66
Woman's Own 92, 93
Working Woman 32, 36

Zinsser, Hans 156